Praise for *Becoming a True Champion*

"After working with great teenage athletes over two decades, I have found a must-read book, *Becoming a True Champion* by Kirk Mango. This book accurately describes a path that teenagers and their parents can follow to achieve greatness in the teen's personal and athletic life."

—**Ken Braid**, cofounder of the
J. Kyle Braid Leadership Foundation

"As young men and women set their sights on a championship, they ask themselves what it will take to become a champion. Kirk Mango provides a clear answer to that question and at the same time takes the concept of 'champion' and extends its meaning into life beyond the athletic arena. . . . Kirk Mango's book should be in school libraries everywhere. His actual experiences as a championship athlete and first-hand knowledge of today's teens as a coach make his advice especially relevant."

—**Mindy Null**, American Library Association
member and high school library department chair

Becoming a
True Champion

Becoming a True Champion

Achieving Athletic Excellence from the Inside Out

Kirk Mango
with Daveda Lamont

ROWMAN & LITTLEFIELD PUBLISHERS, INC.
Lanham • Boulder • New York • Toronto • Plymouth, UK

Published by Rowman & Littlefield Publishers, Inc.
A wholly owned subsidiary of The Rowman & Littlefield Publishing Group, Inc.
4501 Forbes Boulevard, Suite 200, Lanham, Maryland 20706
www.rowman.com

10 Thornbury Road, Plymouth PL6 7PP, United Kingdom

British Library Cataloguing in Publication Information Available

Library of Congress Cataloging-in-Publication Data

Mango, Kirk, 1957-
    Becoming a true champion : achieving athletic excellence from the inside out /
Kirk Mango with Daveda Lamont.
        p. cm.
    Includes bibliographical references.
    ISBN 978-1-4422-1406-4 (pbk. : alk. paper) — ISBN 978-1-4422-1407-1 (ebook)
        1. Sports—Psychological aspects. 2. Sports—Moral and ethical aspects. 3. Athletes—
Psychology. 4. Athletes—Professional ethics. I. Lamont, Daveda. II. Title.
GV706.4.M35 2012
796.01—dc23   2011044671

∞™ The paper used in this publication meets the minimum requirements of American
National Standard for Information Sciences—Permanence of Paper for Printed Library
Materials, ANSI/NISO Z39.48-1992.
Printed in the United States of America

To my daughters, Shaina and Lindsey, who helped inspire me to write *Becoming a True Champion*. It was through their choices and their athletic endeavors that I found genuine purpose behind the need for such a literary piece. Even with the multitude of experiences I had as an athlete, coach, and educator, all of which gave rise to the information in this book, it was through raising my daughters that I found the comfort and encouragement to forge a path toward its completion. So it is with great pride that I dedicate this book to my two girls.

All my love,
Dad

Contents

SECTION III
Putting It All Together—A True Story
177

Foreword

by Nadia Comaneci

$\mathcal{N}$o one really knows when he or she is about to make history. There are no instruction books or lesson plans about how to handle the moment. As I swung onto the parallel bars at the 1976 Olympics in Montreal, I executed each skill with the proper technique—skills that I had diligently practiced day after day in training. Though I performed the same compulsory routine as every other gymnast in the Olympics, I had worked very hard in training to add a little extra "Nadia" touch. I thought my routine had been good, but I knew it was not perfect.

But at the time I didn't analyze my performance. It was done, and I needed to move on and get ready for the next event, the balance beam. While I warmed up for the beam, my score for the bars flashed across the scoreboard. The crowd began to mumble in confusion, for the scoreboard said "1.00." No one knew what "1.00" meant. I continued to warm up, focused on my next routine and unaware of what was happening.

Then the announcer said, "The score for Nadia Comaneci is a perfect 10!" I realized that the perfect score had been given to me because my performance had been better than the previous gymnast, who had earned a 9.95, and the judges had no other choice.

From that moment on, my entire life changed. Even today, more than thirty years later, I am still recognized as the woman who scored the first perfect 10 in Olympic history. Many wonderful

Olympic gymnasts have come and gone since me, but the fact that I was the first to get a perfect score continues to define my life.

More than anything, I learned how much hard work and dedication it takes to be a champion. That is why I am happy to support and recommend *Becoming a True Champion* by Kirk Mango, with Daveda Lamont. A very fine gymnast, Kirk realized that there are many life lessons to be learned from a positive experience in sports. As an athlete, coach, teacher, and parent, Kirk has seen many good—and bad—examples of the sporting experience. He knows there is a big difference between what it takes to simply be "the winner" of a contest and what it takes to be "a true champion." In this book Kirk has taken it upon himself to clarify these concepts for all athletes so that they have the opportunity to reach the highest possible levels of athletic achievement.

Perhaps when I was a competitor it was a more innocent time. These days the stakes are very high, and unfortunately, many people have lost the perspective of the true reasons for participation in sports. Today there are many examples in the media of bad sportsmanship, selfish play, cheating, and the use of performance-enhancing drugs.

Despite the prevalence of these hazards in the sports environment, many important life lessons can be learned through practice and on the field of play. Therefore, at ages where it can make a difference, athletes need to be encouraged and inspired every day by examples of fair play, hard work, good sportsmanship, dedication, and teamwork. This book shows them what all these words really mean, what their importance is, and enlightens them about the real dangers and pitfalls they may confront. In short, it charts a pathway they can follow toward great athletic accomplishment.

I am often asked what the secrets to my success were, and I am always proud to explain that there were no secrets. I was a champion because I worked extremely hard; I had the ability to focus on the keys to success, plus I had the mental strength to tune out the distractions. Most important, I took personal responsibility for my successes and failures. These qualities still serve me well today as a wife, mother, businesswoman, and volunteer for several charities.

But not all athletes are fortunate enough to have mentors and others who can teach them these important attitudes and concepts. This book fills that gap. I am certain that the athletes who study this book and apply what it teaches them will, without a doubt, learn what they need to know and do to succeed in their highest aspirations.

I wish you success, and I hope you score your own perfect 10 in sports, and in life!

— Nadia Comaneci
First gymnast to earn a perfect score in Olympic competition
Five-time Olympic gold medalist

Message to Aspiring Athletes from Phil Wunderlich

There are countless talented young athletes in this world, and it is likely that most of them will come to a point where they are challenged and will begin to question what they thought they knew and what they believed they wanted. Whether during this moment of reckoning, or before it actually occurs, *Becoming a True Champion* is the book athletes need to read because it teaches them to analyze what they are doing and how it is affecting their athletic career.

For me, this moment came about two-thirds of the way through my first season as a Division I baseball player. Baseball has consumed much of my life for as long as I can remember. I had always excelled and never truly faced real, consistent failure in my sport. I received a baseball scholarship to the University of Louisville, and I made a positive impression on my coaches and teammates from the start with my work ethic and through my performance in the off-season scrimmages.

The season came, and on opening day I was in the starting lineup with high expectations from everyone, the highest coming from myself. However, as is sometimes the case in sports, things did not go as I had expected. I suppose the best way to describe my overall performance that first season was "disappointing." And once I started to really struggle, I did not know how to handle it. My mind-set was very poor, and I was just not mature enough to deal with that type of failure. By the end of the season, I was only starting one out of every two games, and baseball had become much less fun. During that season, somewhere along the line, I had forgotten the important lessons I learned from Kirk Mango—the ones outlined in this book.

After such a tough first year, and before my sophomore season, I wanted to make sure that I did everything in my power to be successful. That following summer before the season, I gave some thought to what I really wanted to accomplish, along with the thought processes I would need to get there—the same thought processes that Kirk teaches and encourages in athletes. These were concepts that helped push me forward to work as hard as I possibly could. And with that refreshed sense of commitment, I came back to campus the next September with a whole new mind-set, and as a result I had a good amount of success.

From that time on I have enjoyed the sport I love more than ever. I was an All-American in my sophomore and junior seasons and was an invitee to the USA National Team trials. Then, in June of 2010, everything I had worked for finally paid off when the Tampa Bay Rays selected me in the MLB draft. In my first season of professional baseball I was an all-star and was named the MVP of my minor league team by the Rays.

All of my success as an athlete and individual runs parallel with the messages in *Becoming a True Champion*. The book starts your journey by establishing the proper mind-set from which to grow. This is without question the most important ingredient for success in any aspect of life. The book shows you the path to excellence and continuing achievement. Ultimately, it is up to the athlete to either follow or not follow the right path, but I can think of no better guide for accomplishing that than this book.

Becoming a True Champion goes on to discuss what it really takes in terms of work ethic, conditioning, training, etc., to excel. Everyone thinks they work hard, and most convince themselves of this, but the fact is that one can always work harder, and Section II conveys the exact right knowledge for you to establish this framework. This is where the book truly connects with Section I, for without establishing a proper mind-set, one will not be willing to put in the necessary work and make the needed sacrifices. At this point, some may still doubt the process, believing they do not have the ability or attributes necessary to excel. However, by the end of Section III, there will be no room for doubt.

I found Section III, the story of Kirk Mango's difficult rise to the pinnacle of his sport, nothing short of inspiring. This story will inspire athletes to go from merely *wanting* to make their high school team, receive a scholarship, go pro—whatever their dreams are—to *really believing* they will achieve their goals.

Sports participation is truly unforgiving and at times even cruel, but it is also immensely enjoyable and rewarding. *Becoming a True Champion* is a book that will help athletes learn how to handle obstacles and ultimately enjoy success, because they will have done what is needed to earn that success. It will help them get through that fork-in-the-road "moment" described earlier—the one that makes athletes question and doubt themselves. This is a book I will continue to reference throughout my professional career and life because I know that it is the handbook for true success. I consider it an honor that these words will have a place in the same pages as these masterful lessons. Thank you, Kirk.

—Phil Wunderlich
MLB Tampa Bay Rays draftee

Acknowledgments

$\mathcal{W}$riting any book is an immense undertaking, and *Becoming a True Champion* was no exception. However, I have been fortunate to have wonderful family members and to have encountered many other fine individuals throughout my life who in their own ways have helped inspire, challenge, and support me in my endeavors. Whether it was by giving me direction and encouragement or just by being there when I needed it, all of these people deserve credit for helping turn the idea of this book into reality. My sincere and deepest thanks go to:

My father and mother, Frank and Joyce, who supported me financially and emotionally whenever the need arose, and my brother, Doug, who became my coach, closest friend, and confidant all through high school and beyond. Cindy, my sister, who looked up to me as her big brother and who was always there for support. Coach Llewellyn Iffland, who truly believed in me that final season of my senior year in high school.

Our agent, Linda Konner; our publisher, Rowman & Littlefield; and our editors, Suzanne Staszak-Silva and Elaine McGarraugh, for recognizing the genuine need for this book and for all their hard work to get its message out to aspiring athletes and the parents and coaches who help make their success possible.

Olympic Gold Medalists Nadia Comaneci and Bart Conner for their willingness to read and offer critiques that helped the book come to life, in addition to taking the time and energy to write a great foreword and endorsement despite their busy family and celebrity schedules.

Ken Braid and the J. Kyle Braid Foundation for the endorsement and suggestion that helped enhance the message of the book for all athletes. Professional athletes Steve Weatherford, Phil Wunderlich, Rob Scahill, paralympian and motivational speaker Lloyd Bachrach, library department chair Mindy Null, and Dr. Robert A. Weil for giving their time to read the book and endorse its message.

Brett Ward and Sue Nucci for their reading, review, and endorsement of the manuscript—their experiences as Division I college athletes were of great value.

The student athletes who enthusiastically volunteered to read the book and demonstrate its worth to the multitude of young adult athletes who comprise an important segment of the book's readership.

A very special thanks to Daveda Lamont, my coauthor, whose writing expertise helped to create a book that has timeless value and impact for any athlete, coach, or parent willing to peruse its pages. Not only were her contributions to the substance of the book significant and her editing exemplary, but also the direction she gave me throughout the writing and publication process was truly extraordinary. And to my father, Frank R. Mango, for creating the illustrations that appear throughout the book, and Khanada Taylor for her work in preparing this artwork and the Circle of Achievement for publication.

Finally, I would like to thank my wife, Chris, for all of her help in finding the meaning behind the words and for standing by me when days turned to nights and nights became early mornings as I pushed through creating each chapter in *Becoming a True Champion: Achieving Athletic Excellence from the Inside Out.*

A Champion

— **Champions**—and championship teams—are made, not born. They use their God-given talents to reach their full potential and allow nothing to come between where they are now and where they want to be.

— **Champions** understand and believe that their limitations are governed only by their imagination. They perform and practice with a controlled intensity and never allow failure on any given day to take away from their eventual success.

— **Champions** look at any loss or setback as a tool by which they can learn and motivate themselves to even greater levels of performance. Pity those who belittle or underestimate a champion's ability to bounce back from short-term failures. Those who do will barely have time to notice the breeze made when a champion passes them by. You see, true champions believe that they control their destiny, and luck has little to do with what they *will* accomplish. Discipline, commitment, sacrifice, character, and heart are second nature to them, and they understand that just trying sometimes isn't enough.

— **Champions** want to compete against opponents who are performing at their best and derive much less satisfaction from wins that occur with anything less. They create opportunities for success that would not have occurred without them. True champions are not arrogant, but exhibit a quiet confidence that demonstrates the belief they have in themselves. They know that it is the little things that separate the good from the great and the great from the best.

— **Champions** believe in themselves, not because their coach is good, not because their equipment is good, and not because their teammates are good, but because *they* are good.

Introduction

Sports on the Edge

ARE TRUE CHAMPIONS BECOMING EXTINCT?

Let's face it—what I like to call the "true champion"—honest, true, hardworking, loyal, strong, full of heart, inwardly motivated, incorruptible, and able to pull his or her team out of the worst possible dilemma through sheer will and grit—may be in grave danger of disappearing. This is the kind of athlete who *not only* reaches high levels of performance and achieves many awards, but who also lives by a personal code of conduct that demonstrates an inner excellence *all* can look up to. Unfortunately, if current trends continue, the true champion may one day, not too far into the future, be relegated to the dusty halls of fame as an impossible superhero—someone who was "too good" to be real and never really could have existed— someone you might only see in fiction.

Are the idea and the *ideal* of a true athletic champion no longer relevant to today's impossibly fast-changing world of sports? Are the traditional moral, ethical, and disciplinary values embodied in the idea of a true champion no longer valid? Have peer pressure, political correctness, and raw ambition become the values of the future? And is this the way it should be?

To that I reply "no!" However, it's clear that the actions of too many athletes, amateur and pro, on and off the playing field, demonstrate that this is the trend. While the number of athletes has grown tremendously over the years, this increase in popularity has brought with

1

it a potentially fatal loss of perspective and minimized what athletes actually can and should be gaining through their experience in sports.

Unfortunately, well-meaning, "support-giving" individuals in a position to influence the behavior and attitudes of athletes have exacerbated this same loss of perspective. Hoping to improve athletes' chances of success or record another win in the "W" column, these people go about it in the wrong way by expressing attitudes and responding to everyday athletic problems and situations in ways that hurt athletes' chances rather than advance them. These attitudes hold athletes back from achieving the success they are capable of and too often entirely prevent forward progress. Because of these attitudes, many aspiring athletes are unable to attain the necessary drive, motivation, beliefs, and principles that are so valuable to continued success in the athletic arena—not to mention to success in life.

Skills and qualities such as character, integrity, willingness to sacrifice, commitment, proper setting of priorities, and maintaining a strong work ethic—attributes you really need—have all become much rarer. Instead, the gymnasium, field, and stadium have become places where too many athletes learn to blame other people or circumstances for their own inability and failures. Objective, realistic assessment of weaknesses, deficiencies, and even chronic performance problems might have shown the athlete what obstacles needed to be overcome. Instead, such assessment is often sacrificed in favor of smoothing out hurt feelings or providing shallow "feel-good" excuses that usually consist of blaming some external factor or person for the athlete's failings.

As a result, personal responsibility for the achievement of one's own goals has almost been forgotten, and athletes are not learning and absorbing the know-how needed to correct themselves and bring themselves up to championship levels.

Traditionally, you might look to the professional- and elite-level ranks to find someone or something to aspire to. However, many professional and elite-level athletes—those people up-and-coming athletes naturally look up to and strive to emulate—exhibit the self-defeating attitudes and questionable behavior we're describing here. Too many of these athletes lack character and set poor examples. Short-term gratification and shallow, material motivations—preoccupation with fame, fortune, and leading a fast, glitzy, irresponsible, and self-destructive lifestyle—are rampant. There is a pervasive attitude, well publicized in the press, chiefly embodied in the self-centered question, "What's in it for me?"

For amateur athletes, the answer to this question is too often thought of only in terms of money, fame, free merchandise, scholarships, and other benefits, such as ease of scoring with the opposite sex and frequent hard partying. For professionals, it is increasingly clear that the chief motivation, in addition to the shallow, external motivators mentioned in the previous paragraph, is a large paycheck and all the other material add-ons that go along with professional success—not the least of which can be an insolent, arrogant attitude toward their employers and the fans. Among players in some sports, it has become desirable to emulate the attitudes and behavior of thugs and gangs and sometimes to glorify and participate in illegal activities of various kinds. The development of character and integrity alongside athletic achievement is being lost, and it is becoming harder and harder to find professional athletes who meet the definition of what I call a "true champion."

The kind of champions I'm speaking of, the kind I want to inspire you to become, do what they do because they want to be good at their sport. They set good examples by achieving their goals through sweat and hard work, and they look at all the monetary and other external advantages as secondary benefits rather than rights and privileges they feel are owed to them. It is these rarer attitudes and values that bring you real, lasting inner rewards, satisfaction, and happiness. So, in my opinion, choosing to travel in the current direction described here can put you on a very *un*rewarding path—sometimes one that leads to ruin and dishonor, if it extends all the way into illegal or destructive lifestyles. Rather, it is the higher ideals that I would like to encourage you to strive for.

WHAT IS THE RELEVANCE AND USEFULNESS OF THIS BOOK?

This book is badly needed. It shows how the ideas and ideals mentioned above, so little understood and valued today, are not icing on the cake, but very real components and prerequisites of sustained success and championship in every athletic arena. *Becoming a True Champion* is designed to help athletes connect with what these original and traditional values and habits are all about and understand why they are more important than ever to their athletic careers and their entire lives.

Additionally, high school and college athletes need to better understand and take hold of their own personal ownership of—and responsibility for—any objective or goal they seek to achieve. They need to understand what such responsibility has to do with excelling in their chosen sport. These concepts are not new and *should* sound like common sense; however, their use and application have become too rare among today's developing competitors.

And for those athletes who don't yet know what they want to do with their lives, these ideas may inspire them to strive for excellence in their favorite sports activity and to start on a path that can offer them stiff challenges to meet and great personal rewards.

By sharing the information in this book, I hope to help athletes build a strong foundation for success by showing them how to develop these "intrinsic" (inner) qualities that are so valuable to success in life. Only in this way will they learn to understand and realize the unlimited potential they have within. And in so doing, they will create opportunities for themselves that they originally may not have believed were possible.

This is ultimately a much more rewarding and satisfying path than the one so many current athletes are presently following—one that can lead them to the fulfillment of their greatest dreams.

INSPIRATIONS

One method I've used to help inspire and encourage the individuals and teams under my direction has been to write short monologues and poetic essays that emphasize the inspirational concepts I teach. My hope in writing these is to reach inside each athlete and help pull out the true champion and spirit of success that each one possesses.

Six of these works appear in this book. I hope they help you to feel on a gut level the power and importance of the things I teach in *Becoming a True Champion*.

The Code of a True Champion

1 Consistently, and without reservation, strive to reach my **full potential**.

2 Be **committed** and **disciplined** in my approach.

3 Take **personal responsibility**, and any action necessary, to achieve team and individual **goals**.

4 Demonstrate a deep **desire** to succeed, applying **passion** and **heart** to any and every task at hand.

5 Show an **impeccable** and **relentless work ethic** that only true **dedication** provides.

6 Set **priorities**, and make the required **sacrifices**, that enhance the chances for athletic success.

7 **Persevere** through adversity with a **positive attitude** and **concentration** that strives toward **excellence** and **mastery**.

8 Establish a **mind-set** that highly encourages the **belief** and **confidence** that one can accomplish anything, if they are so willing.

9 Apply a **training** and **competitive focus** that creates the opportunity to transform the impossible into the possible.

. . . All set on a foundation of strong **character** and **integrity** that beseeches one to do the right thing just because it is the right thing to do.

And so, you may ask, "Why follow a code of such high standard?"

- Because I believe I can make a difference.
- And because I believe it,
- Then it is something I should do.
- Because it is something I should do,
- Then it is something I *will* do.

So I toil and sweat both through the good days and the bad:

- Chipping away at any weakness that following the code may reveal within,
- Creating inspiration from athletic experiences of days gone by,
- From future experiences that have yet to occur,
- And from those who may someday attempt to walk the same path—
- Never giving up,
- Never giving in,
- And never swaying—but for a moment—from the Code of a True Champion.

Again, one might ask, "Why?"
Simply—**Because *I can!!!***

SECTION I

The Principles of a True Champion— Someone Only in Legends?

*W*hat were your first thoughts when you picked up this book and read the title, *Becoming a True Champion: Achieving Athletic Excellence from the Inside Out*? Did you picture yourself making incredible plays, perfecting difficult skills, or attaining goals that may have eluded you in the past? Did you have feelings of excitement and hope and think you just might have found the answer you were looking for?

If so, that is a great start. If not, those feelings will come. For it is in this first section that you will begin to build the necessary internal foundations that create an opportunity few actually are able to realize. No, it's not something you had to be born with! Anyone with the will to learn new things and put them into practice can do it. The makings of a true champion are not just found in storybooks— they are right inside *you*.

In this section you are going to learn about things that many coaches and teachers today spend little time discussing—things that some people in athletics place minimal value on and don't concern themselves with. It's going to take some courage, and your friends and peers aren't all going to agree with you about these things. Some may give you a hard time about them. We're not going to just talk about how to succeed physically and objectively in athletics, but we'll also discover what your mind and heart have to do with it.

We're going to deal with the intrinsic (inner) qualities and characteristics of a true champion and show you a process that you can follow to greatly improve as an athlete and to reach, maintain, and *improve upon* championship levels, if that is your goal. The overall purpose of this book is to assist you to succeed and accomplish your athletic goals and objectives. I wrote it in a way that will help you to develop *your own* framework (mental plan, structure, or outline) for success. You can take all of the elements and components and use them "out of the box," just as they are written here, or you can adapt them to fit your individual needs as an athlete.

• Chapter 1 •

It Starts with You

Realizing Your Potential
and Creating Success

You are about to take your first steps into the realm of the true champion. It is the start of a journey that will require self-reflection as we go through this process and build, brick by brick, the components you will need to reach your desired level of success in athletics. While I have not as yet discovered any formal research that "proves" what I'm about to teach you, my ideas are based on the firm convictions that my own experiences and successes as an athlete and coach have given me. I have discovered for myself what works, and that is what I want to share with you in this book. So, while you may run across people from time to time who disagree with something I've said or written here, keep in mind that there were also many people who disagreed that I could achieve the stiff athletic goals I set for myself as a junior in high school—and they were as wrong as they could get.

How wrong were they? You'll read in Section III, "Putting It All Together—A True Story," how I took myself from a mediocre gymnast on the still rings event to Illinois state champion in just under a year—a difficult task that practically everyone told me was impossible. I didn't let myself become discouraged or give up. In fact, just having so many people saying I *couldn't* do it helped make me very determined to accomplish my dream—a dream that eventually led to my winning an NCAA Division I National Championship in competition against several Olympians.

THE FIRST LESSON

This is the first lesson—and it is one of the most important ideas in this book: It doesn't matter how many people disagree with what you want to do. The only important thing is what you believe to be true, and the choices you make to realize your goals and dreams. What you then do is your choice alone. In other words:

All real success and achievement result from *your own choices*, not those of others who may try to make your choices for you.

It is essential to understand that *anyone*—that means *you*—can become the champion you dream of becoming—if you truly want it and are willing to take your future into your own hands and make it happen. This is true even when facing very difficult odds or circumstances.

Take, for example, Bethany Hamilton, the surfer who in 2003, at age thirteen, was ravaged by a tiger shark while surfing off the island of Kauai in Hawaii. The attack severed Bethany's left arm and caused her to lose more than half her blood. Just surviving such an ordeal would be tough enough for most people. However, this inspirational young lady not only recovered from this terrible misfortune, but also came back to surf again only one month after the attack! And surf she did, demonstrating outstanding skill in open surfing competitions. She was able to turn her dream of becoming a professional surfer into reality four years later, in 2007. So moving is Bethany's story that her autobiography was turned into a feature-length film titled *Soul Surfer*.[1]

Now, think about how this story relates to the idea of success in sports being tied to one's choices. Do you think that, after her accident, Bethany made the types of *choices* that improved her chances for recovery and increased her odds of coming back to surf again and compete successfully? Was it the choices *she* made that enhanced the probability that she would reach her dream of turning pro?

And how about you? Are you making the kinds of choices that will help you get out of sports what you are looking to achieve? Read on and let's find out!

FUNDAMENTAL PRINCIPLES

The basic qualities of a true champion are developed from within and become a natural part of you, so I refer to them as "intrinsic" fundamental principles (meaning qualities that come from inside you, or those that you consciously develop within yourself).

By the way, it might help to check the meaning of the word *fundamental* here, because it's a very important word in this book.

A *fundamental* is something upon which other things rest and depend.

So when we speak of fundamental principles, we're talking about important basic qualities *you can develop* that will enable you to succeed. They are the building blocks of success for any athlete who wants to excel. They are the motivators behind the effort you put forth. In the absence of the fundamentals we are going to talk about, an athlete is merely "going through the motions."

Many years ago one of my student athletes, a freshman in high school, told me how he was going to be a state champion in wrestling someday. He was a pretty good athlete, and I felt he genuinely had the athletic ability to reach this lofty goal. However, his efforts in my physical education class were very lackluster, and some of the choices he made outside of class didn't come close to the fundamental qualities I will be showing you how to develop in the first section of this book. Needless to say, he never did accomplish his dream of state champion. In fact, it saddens me to tell you that I don't believe he even finished high school—at least not where I taught.

The word *fundamentals* has another meaning relating specifically to sports and athletics. It refers to *the most basic and primary elements and skills of any sport or athletic activity*. It can also mean *the basic movements of any specific skill or trick an athlete performs.* So in baseball, throwing and catching are fundamentals. In volleyball, underhand and overhand passing are fundamentals. In gymnastics, a handstand is a fundamental. More on this later.

THE DIFFERENCE BETWEEN
A CHAMPION AND A TRUE CHAMPION

Again, there are some who will maintain that not all of the principles I present are essential for championship performance. They will bring up many examples, both in amateur and professional athletics, where individuals did not demonstrate the attributes I name as fundamental yet are still considered great athletes. Well, I would agree that those people are great athletes—but they are not necessarily great or true *champions*.

You can clarify this point further for yourself by answering the following question. How often do you hear of scandalous behavior exhibited by some very accomplished athletes—even great athletes? Based just on what we've covered here, would you consider them *true champions*?

As you can see, I do not define the "true champion" just as someone who wins or breaks records. The way athletes act, what they stand for, and what they do *off* the field are all as important as what they do on it. True champions live their life based on certain principles, and it is these principles that distinguish them from other athletes. (There are also a few principles we'll cover that, while not essential to becoming a true champion, are still extremely helpful in creating an environment for success.)

Here's another pretty amazing thing. *Following these same principles actually makes possible the achievement of goals that others believe are impossible*—even that you may initially believe are impossible. Following them allows the true champion to transcend life's apparent limitations and barriers and achieve success—even against tremendously steep odds. And in so doing, the champion creates for himself or herself a true and deep sense of well-being.

SELF-MOTIVATED AND
SELF-CREATED EXCELLENCE

If many of my own most memorable experiences hadn't been connected in some way with athletics, I may never have seen life from my particular perspective or developed the attitudes and opinions I have about achievement in sports. My viewpoint, along with many of the teachings in this book, is based on the idea of self-motivated and self-created excellence. This is the kind of self-motivated and self-created excellence that Bethany Hamilton must have shown in order to accomplish what she did and the kind that the young high school wrestler I detailed earlier was unable to demonstrate.

In fact, the extreme workability of this approach helped motivate me to write this book, and it will help you to write your own "story" of athletic achievement.

Through this book, I want to teach and show you that everything you aspire to in life can be had—if you make the right choices and follow the right actions. Most important, I want to show you that each individual is the sole controller of his or her own destiny in their chosen activity.

Now, this is not to say that merely by making the right choices, every athlete will always enjoy success. There are no absolute guarantees, no matter how much time you put in, how hard you work, or how hard you try—because life is not always fair. Everyone encounters obstacles, barriers, and problems over which they have little or no control. But it is the *controllable* aspects that really dictate eventual success—and showing you those is what this book is all about.

EVERY PERSON HAS GREAT POTENTIAL

It is my belief that each and every person has tremendous potential. The key to unlocking this potential lies in your ability, first, to discover the broad areas in which your strongest interests lie—the things you enjoy the most—and then to move toward developing your abilities and talents in those areas. I also believe that true *happiness* results from one's ability to accomplish this. I'm talking about the kind of happiness that allows people to look themselves straight in the mirror and say truthfully, "I like who I am, what I've become, and who I plan to be." This is the kind of happiness that gives a person the confidence and belief that they can accomplish anything they want, if they are willing to work hard at it and persist.

Take a moment or two to think about those things you really enjoy doing. If you happen to have a natural talent in those areas, all the better. Those are the things that you have the most potential in, and they are the things that can eventually bring back to you a deep sense of self-satisfaction when you apply the concepts provided in this book.

TEACHINGS IN SPORTS TODAY

All that said, there can still be many obstacles to an athlete's path to success, in view of the way sports are being taught today. As a high school and college athlete, a teacher and coach, and parent of two daughters who played high school and college sports, I have seen and heard a lot—some good, some bad, and some very troubling. These experiences have shown me the mistaken ideas many have about how athletic success is best achieved. Laboring under such misconceptions will make the obstacles you face that much more daunting. And becoming an accomplished athlete is already a tough road to travel for most; it is that much harder if you are unable to recognize the pitfalls that some of these misconceptions can cause.

I have considered these difficulties for quite some time and found that two powerful concepts, above all, can either positively or negatively influence your ability to succeed in sports.

These concepts are *Responsibility for Success* and *Development of Intrinsic Motivation* (motivation from within).

OK, let's get into what this is all about.

WHO CREATES SUCCESS?

So who is really responsible for an athlete's success? Is it the coach, the parents, the club or team they play for—or maybe the school?

Well, if you listen closely to what some athletes discuss after a loss (and what many spectators talk about on the sideline during games), you would think that any one—or all—of the people and organizations mentioned above are the responsible party rather than the athletes themselves. Yet it has been my observation, over and over again, that the *athlete must shoulder responsibility for his or her own success and that of the team, if they are to excel.* In a team, *all* the athletes share the responsibility—that means they each *individually* must willingly take it and resolve to try his or her hardest to contribute to that success.

To illustrate the truth of this concept with a ridiculous example, imagine a men's basketball team in which half the members said or believed, "I really don't think we can win, because our coach is not very good and the lighting in this gym is too dim for me to shoot effectively. So I guess it's up to the rest of you guys. I'll just play along and do what I can, but don't count on me that much to help us win."

The problem with this attitude is obvious! No one would want to play with these guys, and most athletes would rightfully want them dropped from the team—because they obviously don't think they can make a difference. They're blaming the coach and the gym and aren't willing to take any responsibility themselves for helping the team win—or to even *try* to overcome difficult playing circumstances! They just want a free ride; they want to reap the benefits of winning without having really contributed to it individually.

Even though this is an exaggerated example, it shows what the results would be if too many athletes had this attitude that they "couldn't do anything about it," or if others encouraged such attitudes. Unfortunately, the number of athletes (and supportive individuals) who think like this is increasing.

What's the truth here about who is responsible? Actually, *many* people contribute to the success of any sport or athletic activity, whether it is a team or individual sport. So, of course, outside factors like coaching, parental support, and good programs are going to be important. But it needs to be said more loudly and clearly that the importance of these factors is still *secondary* to the role *you* must play in creating your own success.

Don't make the mistake I have seen so many athletes make by placing the responsibility for their or their teams' success on anything and everything but themselves.

To further demonstrate the inner responsibility you must accept from yourself in order to become a top-notch athlete, let me take you through one experience I had with a parent spectator while watching an athletic event. In this case, it was a high school soccer game and I was there as the parent of one of the athletes, not as a coach.

We were both sitting in the bleachers watching the game. This parent was sitting in front of me. Her daughter had just made several attempts to score but missed the goal widely. She turned to me and said that her daughter's ability to shoot on goal and score had been much better during her club season than it was now during high school. She said that the high school coach needed to give the kids more practice on this skill if her daughter and the team were to improve in this area.

I replied that, even though this may be true, we (meaning we spectators) really need to support the coach's decisions regarding what his athletes practice on, because he may have other priorities for his team that we cannot see from the stands or are just not aware of. Also, he has a limited amount of practice time after school to handle all the needs of the team, so he must set his own priorities. Then I said, "If your daughter is frustrated with her ability to shoot on goal, and score, she might want to take it upon herself to practice that skill on her own."

This mother obviously didn't know what to reply to this, because she just looked surprised and turned her attention back to the game. It apparently hadn't occurred to her that her daughter could step up and take responsibility for her own success.

The bigger, more important question is what you, the athlete, would do if you were subjected to attitudes like the one this parent originally expressed. Would you accept the responsibility for making yourself better, or would you place the responsibility somewhere else? It does not matter where these types of attitudes come from—whether from teammates, friends, spectators, or parents—it is something you will most likely be faced with. What *will* matter is how you respond to it.

JUSTIFICATIONS, ACTIONS, AND ATTITUDES THAT LEAD TO EVENTUAL FAILURE

In today's sports environment, the common philosophy is completely backward. Far too many athletes place the major responsibility for their success on anything and everything except the one person who should accept it—themselves. Let me give you some examples of the types of excuses I've heard, and you have probably also heard:

- blaming the coach for any and/or every loss, for playing the wrong players, or for placing an athlete on a lower-level team (at their high school or club);
- blaming the referee for just about everything that goes wrong;
- keeping a mental tally on the number of times certain teammates start, compete, or the amount of time they play and using this to claim unfair treatment (in other words, implying that an athlete's failings are the coach's fault for not allowing them to play enough);
- repeatedly jumping from one club or program to another because the athlete couldn't get what he or she wanted. (This occurs most often because of an issue with playing time, starting position, or player position. It almost always centers around what the athlete wants, instead of what the coach feels to be best for the athlete and team. Ultimately, again, it boils down to blaming every other factor besides an athlete's performance for his or her problems.)
- blaming the coach for not enough practice, too much practice, not practicing the right things, and other supposed failings;
- the gym, equipment, and/or fields are not good, too small, too big, or badly taken care of, which supposedly did not allow the team (or individual) to perform well;
- countless other similar justifications for poor performance.

You should be able to see that most of these items are simply excuses for an athlete's underperformance—they are justifications and rationalizations. Some are clever, some even contain perhaps a small element of truth—but all are quite transparent. This type of behavior is nothing more than playing a "blame game." Blame everything and anything you want except the person who has the most control over changing it—*you*, the athlete.

Let's dig down a little and explore why this is so bad. All of these excuses in some way *remove the major responsibility for success from the competitor and place it somewhere else.* Yet the last time I checked, it is the *athletes* who are on the field of play or in the competitive arena! They, and no one else, comprise the most important factor in determining a win or a loss, a success or a failure. You've probably heard the term *empowering.* Well, making excuses and justifications alleging that various factors besides yourself are responsible for your success or failure is the exact opposite of that—it is *un*empowering, to coin an awkward term! Little by little, such an attitude and practice can rob you of the will and ability to create your own successes.

This is not to say that a coach does not bear some accountability for how the team and individual players perform, based on the correctness of his or her game or training strategy. However, by blaming a *strategy* entirely for a loss, many athletes are persuading themselves that something *outside of themselves* caused the loss. This completely negates the athlete's responsibility for anything that happened in the game and even during practice sessions leading up to competition. And it denies the fact that your own *individual determination and effort can overcome almost any odds.*

ADDITIONAL CONSEQUENCES OF RELYING ON JUSTIFICATIONS

Whether you realize it or not, there is a further cost to both you and your teammates if you adopt the types of justifications discussed above as your own. This idea of placing responsibility for what happens outside of yourself can have a devastating effect on athletes:

It destroys their motivation for trying to do better next time. They think, "Why should I continue trying as hard as I can, if the coach is going to ruin everything with a bad strategy?" Such justifications say, in effect, that no matter what you do or how hard you try, you are powerless to win.

But this thinking is faulty from the word *go* because you can always do better, make a difference, and help to create some level of success, or a win, even against terrible odds—and it is rare that any coach's decisions are as bad as many try to make them out to be. If you use such justifications, you destroy or undermine the *motivation* for doing better, and in doing so, you greatly diminish personal and team athletic potential because you've taken away any reason for continuing to work hard in order to improve.

The other thing that this kind of criticism of the coach does is also very detrimental: it undermines the whole concept of teamwork. A team is a group of individuals working together and supporting each other to achieve a goal. If athletes' confidence and trust in their team leader—the coach—is weakened or destroyed, then the athletes have lost their best source of guidance in the sport and they have been robbed of their ability to function as a smooth component of a unified team. This would only be justified by extremely serious or repeated destructive behavior on the part of a coach—serious enough to warrant a formal complaint. So you should really think hard before you tear down the coach—the negative impact this can have for you and the team you play for is far-reaching. Know your stance going in and make sure you become part of the solution and not part of the problem, as detailed above.

TIME TO MAKE SOME DISTINCTIONS

It is very possible you are starting to feel the weight of personal responsibility for your own athletic success being thrust on your shoulders. That is certainly an important aspect of any athlete's, or any person's, ability to learn how to take charge of their own destiny and become successful. However, it is important that I make some distinctions between your role as the athlete and the role of others.

It is not my intent to remove the normal responsibilities other important people in your life may have in supporting your efforts. It would be a grave mistake for you to think or act in a manner that negates their significance to your success. Taking a position that it is "*all* up to the athlete" is *not* what I mean when I say that athletes must learn to take responsibility for their own achievement. There are *many* people who will contribute to your success as an athlete. A perfect example is your coach—his or her role of training and guidance is essential. This is also true of your parents' role of supporting you. But parents and coaches cannot take your place and somehow "make up the difference" if you never realize and *follow through on your own ability and responsibility to create athletic success.* Showing how *you* can do this is the subject of the rest of this book.

Conversely, you could make a good argument for the idea that a coach should put in as much effort and energy as the athletes do—perhaps more. After all, the best coaches and teachers are the best because they serve as the best living example of what it is they are trying to teach. The same can be said about parents. However, these are aspects over which you really have no control. I want you to remember something I said earlier in this chapter: *It is the controllable aspects that you want to concern yourself most with.* They are the things that will ultimately determine your level of success. And those controllable aspects—they center on *you.*

MEETING CHALLENGES VERSUS PLAYING THE BLAME GAME

In order to bring about a deeper understanding of how important it is to take charge of controllable aspects—which helps you meet challenges—and stay away from blaming others, let's take a look at Paul the soccer player.

Paul plays for a well-respected club soccer team not too far from his hometown. He is a very skilled player whose competitiveness gives him an edge. However, Paul seems to have some difficulty accepting the referee's calls (rulings) during games. Obvious ones are not a problem; it's the close ones that go against him or his team that Paul goes ballistic over. His reactions are negative, sometimes verbal, and it affects his game, as Paul's skill level drops any time he perceives a "bad" call. And whenever his team loses, Paul's most often used statement, "If it wasn't for that ref!" is clearly audible to anyone nearby.

Do you know anyone like Paul? Ever hear that statement before? It is certainly one of Paul's favorites. However, what Paul has not realized here, and what *you* must realize, is that whether a referee, judge, or umpire was bad or not is irrelevant, because *you have no control over him or her, and focusing on what that other person did takes attention away from your own responsibility in the game.* It certainly did for Paul.

Obviously, having to contend with an unfair referee is not fair—but it is part of the learning process for an athlete to figure out *how to rise above adversities that he or she has no control over—even those that are not fair.*

And there is something else about our talented soccer player Paul. He has played on four different traveling teams in the last three years, moving from one to another whenever things did not quite go his way. Yep, our friend Paul doesn't ever settle in anywhere for too long, as there always seems to be something "not fair" at every club he has ever played for. I refer to what Paul is doing as *club jumping,* and it has become a common occurrence these days.

Jumping to another club team or club program is one more way of trying to avoid or get around the normal challenging obstacles that athletes need to overcome in order to truly benefit on all levels from their participation in sports. The grass is *not* always greener on the other side of the fence.

That does not mean there is never a reason for an athlete to change programs. If you were truly being mistreated in some way, or the program lacked a sense of discipline (the kind needed to develop your character), or it simply did not help with your "complete" athletic development (your physical, mental, emotional, social, and fundamental needs), then it may be time to move. However, what is essential for you to keep in mind is that the move must be dictated only by what is in your "real" best interest as an athlete. More times than not, the change in program is being prompted by an obstacle that the athlete wants to avoid or get around or believes is unfair. Often, this obstacle is not getting enough playing time. Well, as I've stated, life is not always going to be fair, and guess what, neither is playing time—especially for the competitive athlete.

My perspective on playing time is simple. If you are not getting all the time that you want, then you, the athlete, had better take the steps to *improve* so that the coach realizes that he or she cannot succeed *without* you in the competitive arena! If you think about it, it is unlikely that any competent coach would give more playing time to players of lesser ability on a consistent basis. So the key is for *you*, the competitor, to attain the skills, techniques, and strategies needed to make the team better!

If you feel you're not getting enough practice or not practicing the right things, then what would be wrong with you, the athlete, putting in extra time on your own to accomplish what you want? If it's always "someone else" or "something else" that caused a problem—then *how can a competitor ever develop their own inner motivation, when "nothing" is ever their fault or responsibility*? And how likely is it really that *nothing* the athlete experiences is his or her own fault? You can see that that is not at all likely. Herein lies my second area of concern, the development of intrinsic motivation.

MOTIVATION FROM WITHIN

Intrinsic motivation is dominated and controlled by our wants and desires, and it is something that is sorely lacking in many athletes today. What do I actually mean by "intrinsic motivation"?

Let me spell this out a little further for you. The word *intrinsic* means "essential" or "belonging naturally," and it originally meant "interior, inner." So intrinsic motivation is an essential, natural inner motivation that the athlete develops and experiences. It is part of the athlete and what makes him or her strive for success.

I would like you to think a little about why there seems to be a lack of inner motivation in so many athletes today. I am sure you have seen this before, maybe among your friends—even some who are very talented athletes. Could it be the fact that so many athletes tend to blame their lack of success on something outside of themselves, as we have been discussing, and thus feel they have little control? Obviously, this is a major contributor; however, it is not the only factor. What about outside pressure placed on competitors by others who put winning as the number-one (or only) priority? It is not unheard of for coaches to punish athletes when they do not win. Additionally, some parents will withhold attention, get angry, or remove privileges when their child is not successful.

You may have experienced situations like this and know how this feels, even after trying your best. For example, have you ever played what you felt was an "awesome" game where everything clicked for both you and your teammates, but you still *lost the game*? And afterward, your coach made everyone run laps because of the loss, or maybe your parents seemed angry with you and you didn't understand why. Whether you are familiar with this situation or not, I am sure you can guess what might happen to an athlete's level of *drive and self-motivation to excel* after experiencing this treatment, especially if it happens on a regular basis.

Now, this is not to say that a parent, coach, or even the program you play for shouldn't have high (but reasonable) expectations for athletes, and it's also not to say that a coach should not institute consequences for poor effort, improper behavior, or not accomplishing performance goals at practice. Remember that these people have a role to play also, and this is a big part of their role. It *is* just to say that you, the athlete, need to be aware of the difference between encouragement that will make you better and misguided discouragement through outside pressure.

Encouragement will help you develop a strong work ethic (the kind that inspires sufficient effort for training and performance), good sportsmanship, teamwork, perseverance, a positive attitude, and other such helpful qualities. These intrinsic qualities are what athletes should hold in high regard, what you should hold in high regard, and many are qualities I talk about in greater detail in later chapters.

As an athlete, you may be asking yourself why any of this is important to know when much of what we are describing here centers on individuals outside of yourself. This certainly falls into the category of aspects over which you have little control. That can be answered with just one word, *perception*! You see, even though you don't have control over a misguided expectation someone may place on you—like "winning" as the number-one priority above all else—and even though you also don't have control over the consequences that may occur for not meeting this expectation, you *do* have control over your perception of that situation, and thus, your attitude about it.

What is important for you to realize here is that, while these responses can inhibit or even crush your drive and self-motivation to excel in your sport, *this can happen only if you allow them to.*

So instead of letting circumstances outside your immediate control get you down, look at them as just another obstacle for you to overcome or another opportunity to improve. Doing so will just make you stronger, and keeping a positive attitude like this, no matter what cards you've been dealt, will be an important factor in your quest to achieve athletic excellence.

OBSTACLES TO INTRINSIC MOTIVATION

I want to discuss with you something that seems to become more prevalent as time passes and which I believe stands as a big deterrent to the development of the internal motivation you are going to need to attain the level of true champion. It is the idea that athletes need to be given some type of external reward for doing well in sports.

I want you to think back to when you were a very young athlete—back to the time when you were playing sports simply because it was fun and you just liked doing well. As you think back, can you recall some of your teammates talking about how they got money or other *external* incentives and rewards for scoring points, goals, baskets, and other similar feats? Now I want you to think about what can happen when an athlete's inner drive to do well (purely for the good feelings they get from doing so) starts to shift into a desire to do well so as to receive that external reward. Would that tend to enhance or diminish the purity and strength of one's inner "will" to do their best? I am sure you know the answer to that.

Personally, I cannot believe the number of times I have seen or heard of athletes receiving external incentives like money, privileges, or much more expensive items such as cars, to accomplish something that athletes *should* want to do just because *they would like to do well* (an intrinsic reason). But the fact is that the more desirable internal motivations can be overshadowed by the "glitz" of external rewards—something I discussed in the introduction. Instead, what athletes, and what you, need to recognize and focus on are the *inner rewards* that develop just through accomplishing something that was difficult.

There is a tremendous feeling of pride and accomplishment that comes from you doing your best. These inner rewards remain with you for the rest of your life, giving you self-confidence, power, endurance, the willingness to work hard toward a goal, and the knowledge that you can accomplish whatever you set your mind to. Can anybody say that about the five-dollar bill an athlete received for scoring a goal?

ARE EXTERNAL REWARDS ALWAYS BAD?

Now, I don't want you to think that accepting external rewards is *always* a bad thing. It would be hypocritical for me to say or imply this. For example, there are many athletes who set the goal of attaining a college scholarship. I was one of them. The key, however, is to keep your center of focus on everything you are doing to accomplish your *long-term goals*, rather than on incentives or rewards for meeting short-term goals like scoring points or winning a game. As long as *you set the goal* and it is only attainable through months and/or years of dedication, sacrifice, and hard work, then a reward for such efforts is definitely warranted and acceptable.

What's the difference? The difference is huge. Taking rewards for a short-term goal *makes the reward the reason for an athlete to put forth effort*. This is *extrinsic* (outside) motivation, and it tends to reinforce itself. It *does not* encourage the long-term process, the improvement of abilities, values, or character, or other long-term development that the athlete should experience. Instead, an athlete is encouraged, and learns, to put forth his or her best efforts only when the reward is external. Remove the reward, and there goes the effort. This is not something you want to set yourself up for.

An aspect you personally may have had the displeasure of experiencing is how detrimental this can be in a team sport. Athletes who are externally motivated like this tend to behave selfishly in the competitive arena. They tend to make decisions based only on themselves and not on the team's needs or goals. There is an old cliché that holds very true here:

There is no "I" in "TEAM."

THE SHORT-TERM GRATIFICATION TRAP

Another significant problem that short-term external motivators cause is how they support the overall trend toward short-term gratification so commonly seen in our society today. Whether it's a crazy new piercing, tattoos, or brand new cars that your friends are given to drive around in, it doesn't really matter. All tend to support short-term gratification with no long-term commitment, discipline, or sacrifice of anything. Therefore they *seriously distract an athlete's attention from what is important.*

It is much harder for anyone to get straight A's, be a great violinist, chess player, cheerleader, baseball player, basketball player, volleyball player, or soccer player and gain attention and respect through those efforts than it is to pierce your eyebrow, get a tattoo, or dye your hair blue and get attention that way. The last three require none of the intrinsic components mentioned above (commitment, discipline, and sacrifice), nor any genuine effort whatsoever, and they bring nothing of real value back to individuals other than the attention they are so desperately seeking.

Therefore, when you engage in such behavior instead of focusing on the intrinsic motivations I have been speaking of, it takes away from what you could and should be learning and acquiring through participation in sports. Any athlete, including one heading for championship, needs to be able to see past this in order to develop to his or her full potential. You really need to stay focused on what you want to achieve and stay away from prioritizing things that bring no *real, lasting* value to you personally or athletically.

As you've begun to discover through this first chapter, this book's purpose is to give you a valid foundation—a workable basis—for success in sports, described in a simple way that will help you attain your own athletic goals. If you take these principles and guidelines to heart, you may find that this foundation also extends above and beyond your success in athletics to help you achieve success in life.

• *Chapter 2* •

Do You Know Where You Are Going?

Goals—The Choice Is Yours

$\mathscr{B}$efore you can travel a path, you must first decide where you want to go. This is why a goal is essentially the starting point for any athletic achievement, as well as the ending point reached after all the work is done. You must decide what you want to accomplish before anything else can be planned and developed. Goals give purpose and direction to everything an athlete is going to do. Without them, a competitor is only playing the game, not deeply *experiencing* or *living* it.

By *experiencing* and *living* your sport, I mean that you are able to draw deeper meaning from and through what you are doing, because goals give you a purpose to live out. Goals that you truly expect to achieve force you to make choices that keep you on a path toward that goal, thus allowing a deeper, richer experience. You are "living" a part of your life through, and as a result of, the direction that your goal has given you.

Without goals, a sport becomes just something you are doing, like going to the movies, browsing the Internet, or going bowling—just something that occupies your time. And for some that is fine—but you should realize that you will not gain as much as you could out of your experience in sports, or from *any* experience, if that is the only way you approach it or look at it.

To better understand what I mean, think about Bethany Hamilton for a moment, the young surfer who lost her arm to a shark but still accomplished her goal of becoming a professional surfer. Do you think she was living a part of her life through her goal, or was it just something she was "doing"? Did she gain deeper meaning through this experience?

WHAT IS A GOAL?

A goal can be very specific, such as a goal to win a state or national title. Or a goal can also be quite general, such as "to be the best you can be" at your sport or activity.

Moreover, goals can be short-term in nature, as in more immediate objectives important for the achievement of future goals. They can also be long term, as we have already discussed. Our main focus here will be on these long-term goals, for they define *your* direction—that place you want to go!

Major league baseball pitcher Jim Abbott's aspiration of becoming a major league pitcher, which I will discuss more thoroughly in the section below on "Creating Goals," is a perfect example of this concept of a long-term goal. Other examples might include winning an athletic scholarship to play your sport at the college level, becoming an All-American or national champion, or even becoming an Olympic champion.

However, goals do not always have to be of this magnitude. Your goal might be just to make a high school athletic team. Or it might be to be the best on your team, the best in your school's conference, or possibly even to place in state competitions.

Personally, I like the idea of making your primary goal one in which you strive to be the best you can be. A goal like this puts control over what happens directly into your own hands because it deals with your own individual potential. No one is in a better position to know, determine, and *expand* your individual potential than you yourself.

Striving to achieve this general kind of goal (to be the best you can be at your sport) helps you concentrate your attention on the real task at hand rather than on less important external factors such as beating out a certain competitor, achieving a certain score, winning a particular competition, or even just the general goal of "winning."

Rather, it spurs you to work on all the things that you need to concentrate on at every practice and every game so as to produce the *improvement* that bit by bit adds up to attaining your long-term goals.

On the other hand, making "winning" the number-one goal, above all else, is a very common mistake made by athletes. The problem with it is that it places the primary focus on your opponent and on what he, she, or they are doing, and therefore puts too much of your concentration on the game or competition itself. Basically, it restricts your vision to *only what it takes to defeat your opponent* and distracts you from what you should be doing at practice to reach your *highest* level of performance now, and as you progress into the future. Therefore, it limits your potential—period! Is this really what you want? (I go further into this point in chapter 7, "A Championship State of Mind," under the heading "Winning and Losing.")

The specific types of goals mentioned above—winning a particular competition, beating the score of one of your competitors, or even achieving a certain score—are extrinsic in nature. Rather than being your own inner-motivated goals (something that you decide upon *before* you compete, to set your future direction), these extrinsically motivated objectives actually are more properly looked at as the *outcomes* or *results* that an athlete achieves through hard work, effort, and proper focus. Concentrating your efforts on the *process*—the work and practice leading to bettering your strong points and improving your weak points—should always take precedence over focusing on outcomes.

Now this does not mean, by any means, that you should not strive to reach extrinsic levels of performance or use them as an objective measure of progress—that is, after all, the purpose of scores and statistics. But it does mean that these extrinsic goals need to be kept in the right perspective and always pursued *in combination with* achieving your ultimate possible potential. Potential, or in this case, athletic potential, is an intrinsic component, and any time an athlete can place more focus in areas that are intrinsic, it is a good thing. This way, win or lose, athletes can always fall back on the fact that they really did the very best that they could in any competition.

Striving to reach your potential is a never-ending struggle, and it gives another advantage to athletes who use this as their primary goal. It has been my experience that your potential *increases* as you improve and move toward it. Other levels of success and performance also open up during this quest. In fact, strangely enough, anyone's potential or potential level of success actually appears to be *unlimited*—at least within the confines of genetic and/or human potential. Remember this:

The higher you set your goals, the higher your achievement.

When setting goals, it is also very likely that you will create a combination of goals in which one goal is dependent upon another. Say you wanted to be the best on your team and get a scholarship to play at the collegiate level. Let's also say that the team you compete for has some of the best athletes in the state, all of whom would normally go on to compete in college on scholarship. Accomplishing being the best on your team will thus most likely also bring with it the goal of the scholarship you are seeking. However, if your team is not very good, yet you want to win a scholarship, you will need to look elsewhere than your team for an appropriate measure of your performance. (In other words, if you only tried to be the best out of a lot of mediocre athletes, you might not be good enough to win the scholarship. You need to find other, better athletes against whom you can judge your performance.)

DON'T BECOME AN OBSTACLE

I want to take a moment here to describe an attitude that can lessen an athlete's willingness to work uncompromisingly toward his or her own athletic goals. This one may be a little harder to spot in yourself and overcome because it appears to stem from the camaraderie and friendship you feel toward your teammates. To illustrate what I mean, let me tell you about Jenny.

Jenny is a very good volleyball player with a lot of potential. Her capability seems open-ended, as she learns quickly, works hard, has a genuine talent toward volleyball that not too many have, would like to become as good as she can, and wants to play at the next level—college. Jenny is also very well liked. Her bubbly personality helps her connect closely with her teammates. She has made strong friendships on the team, something she cares deeply about.

However, it is this same connection to her teammates that also impacts her improvement because she feels reluctant to greatly surpass her friends in athletic ability. She just doesn't want to "show them up" on the volleyball court. As a result, Jenny holds herself back a little and doesn't really go all-out for her goal of becoming as good as she can be. She doesn't want to get *too* much better than her team members or exceed their collective skill level, so she figures she will just improve to the point of being one of the best on the team and then coast along at that level. What Jenny is really doing is acting on a self-generated form of peer pressure—she's actually placing this *on herself* in a wish to fit in with her teammates, even though nobody has said anything to her about it.

You should realize that if you assume this type of attitude, you are placing a "cap" (upper limit) on your improvement and you will stifle your movement toward the goal of being the best you can be. The main thing you need to recognize here is that continually moving toward your personal goals, and not limiting your achievement in any way, is the very *best* thing you can do for your teammates. Not only will you help your team in the best way possible—by becoming better and better—but you will, without even trying, serve as a great example of what can be achieved and very likely inspire some of your friends to do the same.

GOALS FOR IMPROVEMENT

In addition to setting goals like the ones we've discussed so far, which will require you to address the mastery of your strengths (strong points), you will also want to set goals that address improvement of your weak areas or weak points. Obviously, at some point, you'll have to give some thought to both of these areas in order for you to set your goals for improvement. This concept of understanding both strengths and weaknesses is further developed in chapter 7,

"A Championship State of Mind," under the heading "Knowing Your Strengths and Weaknesses."

THE GREATEST LESSON

When you start looking at your training and competitions in the way we've been discussing, you learn one of the most important lessons there is—*you learn to compete only against yourself.* This is an attitude all competitive athletes should try to develop. In my opinion, it is what allows an athlete to reach championship level and then to stay a champion at the highest levels of competition. Once an athlete has reached the top, this will be the key to staying there—by surpassing his or her own highest level, and doing so again and again.

In order to become a true champion, always keep this in mind:

The moment you become complacent (satisfied) with your level of performance is also the exact moment you have forgotten where you were going.

CREATING GOALS

The impetus for a goal can come from just about anywhere. It may come from seeing someone else perform or compete. Admiring the accomplishments of another individual can be a great place to start. It is also conceivable an athlete might want to emulate the characteristics or qualities of several different athletes.

Maybe what you want to accomplish starts with the love you have for your sport (something very common to successful athletes), or from a need to succeed, or a talent you have, or a strong desire to compete, or, most commonly, a combination of all the above.

Whatever the case, the key to setting goals is in looking *beyond* your reach and *beyond* what others may think is attainable, for what others think really has little to do with what can be accomplished.

Do not be afraid to dream big. Taking a risk is part of the game, and nothing worthwhile was ever accomplished by playing it safe.

JIM ABBOTT

What would you think if a young baseball player said his goal was to play in the major leagues? Tough, right? Only a small percentage of ballplayers are ever good enough to make it to the majors. However, Jim Abbott was a young ballplayer who was really special—he had only one hand. What do you think his odds of making it into professional baseball would be, now that you know that? Pretty slim, I'm sure, and you would not be alone in thinking that.

Jim was born on September 19, 1967, with a significant birth defect: his right arm ended just above the wrist. For many, just dealing with the adversity of having one hand, when almost everything in the world around you was designed for people with two, would be tough enough. But Jim Abbott had dreams. He loved playing baseball and wanted to become a big-league ballplayer. When asked about major leaguers who had been an inspiration to him, his response was, "I look at them and wish it were me."[1]

On Saturday, April 8, 1989, he turned his desire into reality. That was the day that Jim Abbott first walked out to the mound to pitch for the California Angels in his major-league debut. Jim spent ten years pitching for outstanding teams in the major leagues, including the New York Yankees, Chicago White Sox, and Milwaukee Brewers, along with the California Angels.[2]

He fulfilled his dream of playing in professional baseball and accomplished his goal.

The message here is that no matter how difficult or impossible a goal may look from the outside, what really counts is what you believe you can accomplish on the inside. Just keep this in mind:

Big dreamers don't always accomplish big things; however, big accomplishments always come from big dreams.

MORE ABOUT SETTING GOALS

Make sure to be realistic about yourself (understand the level of your current skills), understand where your talents lie (so you can use them to your advantage), and know what time frame you have in which to accomplish your goal or goals. It would be foolish to assume an athlete can go from average to great in a week or even a month—common sense dictates the opposite.

On the other hand, it is important to be careful when you use common sense to set and plan the achievement of your goals. Sometimes common sense does *not* apply. Take the U.S. Hockey team's performance over the Soviets in the 1980 Winter Olympics—a victory selected as the greatest moment in sports of the twentieth century by *Sports Illustrated*.[3] Who would have thought that a bunch of young, less-experienced hockey players could come together, challenge, and defeat the USSR on the way to winning Olympic gold! And this was after being trounced by the Soviets in a pre-Olympic exhibition game 10–3. At that time, the USSR had the best hockey team on the planet. Common sense would have said this was impossible—yet it happened.

I am sure if you look hard enough, examples like this abound in every sport and at every level. Don't allow too much "common sense," or too great a reliance on what seems possible or realistic, to limit your achievements! Whatever your goal, always keep in mind that its accomplishment will be much more dependent on what you are willing to *do* to accomplish it, rather than the nature or size of the goal itself.

CLIMBING THE LADDER

To become accomplished as an athlete you will need to be truly invested in your goal (committed to it) since, for the most part, as mentioned before, goals tend to be long term in nature. You also have to create sufficient push and motivation to carry yourself through over a long period. This idea of a long-term investment for most goals can become problematic for you, the developing athlete, because of the distance between your present level and where you expect or want to be. There are always intermediate steps you need to take or plateaus you need to surmount as you progress toward what it is you want to achieve. These steps, or plateaus, are best thought of as intermediate objectives that you set, or obstacles that you overcome, as you practice the skills you need to master in order to be successful in your sport.

Athletes can easily become discouraged if they are continually looking beyond these intermediate steps and thinking about how far away they are from their ultimate goal. Therefore, it is important to take things one little step at a time. Each small step up to a different plateau represents a small step forward toward your goal. Like climbing a very long ladder, you should focus more on the accomplishment of each step up the ladder and much less on what is at the top.

To further clarify, these objectives and obstacles (steps or plateaus) are usually smaller in nature than a goal, but *essential to its successful achievement.* They may encompass things like moving up in the batting order, as in baseball; moving to a starting position in a team sport; or winning smaller competitions before the big event at the end of a season. They may also include things like learning new skills, techniques, or strategies; scoring higher or decreasing one's times as the year passes; moving past competitors or teammates who were better; increasing one's strength and conditioning; or just improving slightly each and every day.

Whatever form they take, what is important is that you take great pride in accomplishing these smaller objectives and overcoming the obstacles. It is these little steps forward that allow you to shorten the distance between you and your goal. I cannot emphasize this concept enough—looking at training this way takes the "im" out of impossible.

GREAT PEOPLE

Great people measure themselves based on what they must do to accomplish what they want, not on what others do. Convincing yourself that you are doing your best because you do more than most, when you are basing your ability and

work ethic on what the average person is doing, will make you just that. Average.

TAKING ACTION
What about Your Goals?

Now that you have read about goals—what they are and how they are used—practice applying them to yourself.

1. Get a piece of paper and pen, or get on the computer. Take a moment or two to think about what you want to achieve in your sport. Think about things that you want to accomplish in the near future—say, *during* the coming season—and also about things that you would like to accomplish in seasons to come. Write these short-term and long-term goals down.

2. Now, let's take this one step further. Reorganize (reorder) your lists so you put the goals in the order in which they should be accomplished, with the ones to be done soonest nearer the beginning. You have now prioritized your goals. The goals nearer the beginning of your list would be considered more short-term goals, with the others being more long-term in nature.

At this point you should be able to see some connection or relationship between the accomplishment of your short-term goals and achievement of your long-term goals—at least with most of them. Getting the short-term goals done should make it possible to do the long-term ones!

If this relationship doesn't appear, you may not have given enough thought to your short-term goals. Take some concentrated time to think of more short-term goals to add to your list; then see if this connection starts to show up.

Save your goals list for upcoming exercises and for future reference.

• *Chapter 3* •

The Burning Within

Desire—The Fuel That Drives You to Move beyond Normal Limitations

*D*o you ever wonder how some individuals and athletes are able to defy the odds? With their chance of success ever so slim, they still seem to find a way to come out on top. Part of the answer to that question is the next step to becoming a true champion.

Once you have determined the direction you want to travel by forming some athletic goals, the next step is to make sure you have—and feel—strong motivation to accomplish these goals and to do the work it will take to achieve them. This motivation will come from, and be directly proportional to, the DESIRE you have to achieve the goals you've set. Athletes with a goal but no desire are often sadly disappointed. They tend to rely on just their talent to get them through, and when things don't go their way, then for them, it all "just boiled down to bad luck." I cannot count the number of times I have heard athletes talk about how good they wanted to be or what they wanted to accomplish, when it was obvious they did not work hard to achieve what they said they wanted. You heard about one such athlete in the first chapter, that wrestler in my class who wanted to become a state wrestling champ but didn't put forth the effort to do so.

What they were sorely missing—what that wrestler did not have—was *desire*. I am not sure I can put into words how important desire is to the motivation of an athlete—to *your* motivation. You really have to *want* to accomplish something in order to have any chance at achieving it. Desire breeds passion, and passion supports, develops, and strengthens *commitment, discipline*, the setting of your *priorities*, and the willingness to *sacrifice* other desirable activities if that is what will make it possible to reach your goals. (I discuss each of these important terms in the next chapter.)

Desire comes from deep within the *heart*—in other words, desire is something you feel very strongly and into which you invest strong emotions. When desire is present, just the thought of *not* accomplishing what you want (your goals) causes some emotional discomfort. Your desire becomes the driving force that develops the determination and perseverance you will need to succeed, and it is what pushes athletes beyond their normal limits, allowing them to set solid priorities, stay on track, and never give up.

Remember the question I asked at the beginning of this chapter? Well, you now have the answer as to how an athlete is able to prepare to beat the odds. The next question is: What will be the source of *your* desire—where will your desire come from?

ADVERSITY AS MOTIVATION

Often a deep determination and desire to excel develops through some sort of adversity that opposes or stands in the way of an athlete's goals, directly or indirectly. The adversity may help focus his or her feelings and desire to succeed in his or her sport. For me (as you will observe in Section III), it took the form of being told that what I wanted to accomplish was not possible, that I was not good enough, that it was too hard, and there was not enough time. That was all I needed to hear, because I was not about to allow *anyone* to predict and attempt to dictate my failure.

For others, adversity might exist in their environment. There are many people, including athletes, who have lifted themselves up out of poverty-stricken conditions, abusive family situations, or other nonsupportive upbringings to achieve great things. Others may have been cut from teams, left on the bench, been seriously injured, been told they were not talented enough, or experienced a previous failure in the athletic arena. Any of these things can spur an athlete on to rise above obstacles and setbacks to excel in sport.

Take James MacLaren, for example. Coming from humble beginnings, Jim was the eldest of three boys and a girl, all of whom had been through a parental divorce and some tough financial times at very young ages. Their family situation forced his mother and stepfather to work very hard in order to provide for the basic needs of their family. Even with this difficult family situation, Jim was able to use his athletic talents, good grades, and the unrelenting support of his mother to secure himself a scholarship to attend Vermont Academy, a college-prep school, to play football. Not an easy task, even for the most privileged! He did so well on the gridiron and in the classroom that he was able to earn a full scholarship to attend Yale University, where he achieved All-American status.

Raising himself out of the *tougher* than average conditions of his childhood might seem enough to prove the important role personal desire plays in overcoming adversity, though some might counter that Jim was just a gifted athlete with plenty of support and was destined to accomplish whatever he set his mind to. They wouldn't have known how severely Jim's desire and will to succeed would be tested in a very short while—not by any stretch of imagination. But for the moment, it looked as if everything was falling into place for Jim and the personal story he was creating.

Jim finished his Yale undergraduate work and relocated to New York City in 1985. Interested in developing his acting career, he was accepted at the Circle in the Square Theatre School on Broadway. Only three weeks later, while riding his motorcycle home late one night from a rehearsal session, Jim was broadsided by a forty-thousand-pound New York City bus in a horrific accident. He was initially pronounced dead on arrival at the hospital. But after eighteen hours of surgery, a comatose Jim was stabilized, and doctors amputated his left leg below the knee.

For many, this would have been all the adversity they could take, but Jim's deep-seated desire and competitive nature did not allow him to merely accept his fate or to embark on a life of self-pity or inaction. He worked very hard through rehabilitation, eventually becoming fit enough to run marathons with the aid of a prosthetic leg. He developed into the fastest single-legged, long-distance athlete in the world. His attitude was exemplified by these statements:

> I felt like I was back in it, back in life. . . . I didn't compete against other people. I was competing against me. A buddy once said, "Mac, nobody cares how fast you go, they just love that you're doing it." I told him I care. I never wanted to be taken for granted, as that guy with the fake leg. So I just kept pushing myself.

Jim's story was well documented in triathlon circles, where, to disabled athletes everywhere, he became someone to emulate. Not only did Jim compete in some of the most difficult races, like the New York City Marathon and the Ironman Triathlon, but he also regularly finished ahead of 80 percent of able-bodied athletes and set numerous records. His training took him all over the world, and the media sought his amazing story. As an inspiration for all athletes, not just the disabled, he delivered many talks and became a loved and well-respected motivational speaker for sports competitors of all types.

But life is not always fair, and adversity once again caught Jim, this time in a manner unmistakably tougher than any he had yet faced. On June 6, 1993, during the bike leg of a triathlon in Mission Viejo, California, Jim was struck by a van. The force was great enough to send him headfirst into a signpost, which broke his neck and left him paralyzed from the chest down—a quadriplegic.

So what did a man like Jim do when, after his hospital stay was over, he had to rebuild his life once again? Jim did what many might consider impossible and what he himself initially thought might be impossible, given the circumstances. With an inner strength that defied understanding, he chose to get the most out of life. He struggled through tremendous physical and mental obstacles to regain limited use of his right arm. He attended graduate school, earned two masters degrees, and started a charitable organization called the Choose Living Foundation. This foundation yearly inspires thousands facing physical and other challenges to fight through adversity. And Jim did not stop there. As a keynote motivational speaker and life mentor, he continued working to realize his own potential by giving back to those in need of the same.

Even with all that was on his plate and all that had befallen him, he started work toward a PhD. Unfortunately, he was never able to complete his degree study. A serious illness overtook him, and Jim died on August 30, 2010.[1]

There are probably many examples I could have selected that demonstrate how essential *deep desire* is to the success and achievement of an athlete—or any individual, for that matter. However, Jim MacLaren's story shows, like no other I've encountered, the tremendous accomplishments possible in the face of staggering odds, when someone draws forth from deep within himself the intense desire to surmount all obstacles and, in spite of everything, achieve his goals and dreams.

CREATING THE PERCEPTION OF ADVERSITY

A different way strong desire and motivation can be accomplished is to create a *perception* of opposition or adversity between yourself and the natural conditions or barriers that occur in your sport. For example, in subjective sports like figure skating, gymnastics, and diving, a person can perceive the judges as adversaries. They are the ones who ultimately decide who wins or loses, and they are the ones who can take away or give the athlete what he or she wants.

But this perception of opposition is not used as an excuse for failure or not making the grade. It is not used to shift the responsibility for failing elsewhere, as covered in chapter 1. Rather, it is used to spur *yourself* on to achieve your goals. The only control a competitor has over the scores a judge awards is through his or her level of performance, and the only way to take control and increase your level of performance is through *proper training*.

So now you, the athlete, have come full circle: the better your training, the better your performance; the better your performance, the better your scores. In my situation in high school, I took the attitude that I would train *so* hard (allowing me to perform *so* well) that the judge would have no other choice but to give out a good score, or look foolish. The choice was his.

The same principle can be applied in team sports; however, you would regard your opponents on the *other* team as your adversary rather than the judge in the above example. The opposing team members would be the ones standing in your way of success. This, again, can be used for motivation to help you train properly.

Remember that here we are focusing on motivation for training. I believe, for the most part, that success will be dictated by what you do during practice, long before competition even begins. How the coach strategizes for game situations is not really under your control; however, your performance of those strategies are. Whether you are involved in team sports or individual sports, and whether success is based on subjective or objective criteria, the only real control you have is over what and how you train and perform. This is where you must focus and where desire becomes extremely important. It is a concept that, along with other related ideas, will be addressed again as we move along the path of becoming a true champion.

TAKE CONTROL

With all of these types of adversity, you have a choice, an option: to accept the position you are in or to *take control of it by choosing not to accept it.* I firmly and wholeheartedly believe that any athlete who wishes to achieve something—anything—must choose *not to accept the position they are in.* It is this type of adversity that sparks the deep desire and determination to accomplish what you want. Even though the original cause (adversity) may have been external, the resulting emotion is intrinsic and allows the true champion to continue working when all others have left. It will allow you to overcome obstacles others see as impassable and to travel the more difficult path even when all others choose the easier one. As Nobel Prize–winning author George Bernard Shaw (1856–1950) put it:

People are always blaming their circumstances for what they are. I don't believe in circumstances. The people who get on in this world are the people who get up and look for the circumstances they want, and if they can't find them, make them.[2]

WILMA RUDOLPH

Champion runner Wilma Rudolph was a legendary example of an athlete whose desire and unwillingness to accept terrible circumstances in life helped her to overcome incredible odds.

Born prematurely on June 23, 1940, in St. Bethlehem, Tennessee, she weighed in at only 4.5 pounds. During this era, premature babies were not expected to live more than a few days. However, Wilma survived. As a child, she was often sick. She got all the usual childhood illnesses, but at age four she contracted double pneumonia and scarlet fever. After her recovery, her parents noticed that her right leg was crooked and partially paralyzed. The pain was so great that she could not walk normally and had to drag herself around.

She had had polio, a very serious and debilitating disease that crippled and paralyzed many of its victims in those days, before a vaccine had been developed. It was not until age six that Wilma got a metal brace for her leg; attached to her shoe, it helped her to get around better, with the aid of crutches. She underwent a great deal of physical therapy with her parents' dedicated help. It took her two more years before she regained enough strength to walk on her own with just the leg brace and no other support.

The doctors had believed that Wilma would never even *walk* normally, even with the aid of a brace. But she wouldn't accept that. She wanted to play, run, and jump with the other kids on the playground. And that wasn't all—she wanted to participate in sports. Something inside Wilma made her refuse to accept her condition. Then, around age nine, she was able to do what no doctor had thought she would ever be able to do: she took off her brace and walked.

From that time she never looked back. Her competitive nature led her to begin to compete with her schoolmates in many physical activities, and she started beating them and excelling. She became an incredible runner. When she was twenty, she competed in the 1960 Olympic Games and won three gold medals—one for the 100 meter dash, one for the 200 meter dash, and the last for the 400 meter relay. Acclaimed internationally, she became known as the "fastest woman in the world." Not bad for a kid who was never expected to even walk normally![3]

The outstanding thing we can take from Wilma's story is that her determination and unbending will would not let her accept the physical limitations that others told her were inevitable. What she tapped into was her inner strength, and this strength formed a *desire* that carried her through great adversity to the highest levels of her sport. Wilma also demonstrated, as did Jim MacLaren, that physical disabilities can be conquered, overcome, and eliminated through strength, determination, persistence, and hard work.

All of us have some level of strength within our hearts; it's just a matter of believing that it's there and then finding it and using it. As Wilma herself put it,

Never underestimate the power of dreams and the influence of the human spirit. We are all the same in this notion: the potential for greatness lives within each of us.[4]

ENJOYING THE PERFORMANCE
OF SKILLS WELL DONE

Desire is so important to the motivation behind athletic success and the achievement of athletic goals that, if it does not happen on its own, you will need to develop it from within. One of the best ways to create desire in yourself is to learn to really enjoy your own performance of skills well done.

Now, I am *not* talking about the feeling one gets when throwing the winning touchdown or striking out the last batter to win the game (even though those feelings provide great motivation in themselves). I am talking about the actual sensation of the fluidity of the performance of a skill—the feeling you get from being able to perform a skill or group of skills so fluently that it becomes effortless, almost instinctive, and seems to become more of an art form than anything else. This sensation is hard to describe. It feels as though everything moves in slow motion, and your body reacts to the stimulus of the competition automatically. There really aren't too many feelings quite like it. Regardless of whether you participate in a team or individual sport, all involve performance of skills and components that can be perfected to this intrinsic level of execution. A lot of my own personal desire to train centered on this concept—especially as I neared my own athletic potential.

Athletes who learn to revel in this feeling will want to repeat it and improve upon it and in so doing will discover a marked increase in their desire to train. This is where the real enjoyment and fun from participation in athletics should come from. This whole concept is intrinsic in nature, and it can give you a true sense of well-being that can only come from deep inside. It is something I would strongly encourage you to work toward and something I explain further in chapter 8, "Separate yet Related."

★ ★ ★

Whatever the situation that you, the athlete, are faced with, the bottom line will be to find a way to create the desire to motivate yourself toward higher levels of performance, the final result being the achievement of your goals. If all of this seems difficult to do, then keep this in mind: *Great people and great athletes desire to be more and better than they are.* Do you?

TAKING ACTION

More Than Just a Feeling!!!

Part One—Desire. In order to determine the level of your own desire, let us try a little experiment. Make sure you have some undisturbed time to yourself to do this.

1. I would like you to think about the goals you developed in the "Taking Action" section at the end of chapter 2. If you feel it would be best to reread them first, then go ahead and do so. Now close your eyes and visualize yourself accomplishing them. Don't think about these goals as just words on a list, but as real-world action. Try to place yourself in the moment, like a daydream, and really "feel" what it would be like to accomplish each one of them, one by one.

Can you see yourself achieving what you set out to do? What do you feel? Is it pride, a sense of accomplishment, or maybe even a feeling of well-being? If you have any positive emotional response to these thoughts, then you are experiencing the sparks of desire—maybe even more than just sparks!

2. Taking this one more notch up the scale, I would like you to go through the same process of visualizing yourself accomplishing each of your goals, but this time add to your thoughts the idea that you are able to perform any skill or play *to perfection*. Truly visualize yourself mastering the skills of the game as you watch yourself succeed at performing or playing the game in your mind. Feel the ease with which you execute skills. Feel how smoothly and effortlessly your body moves, even under the extreme pressure you can artificially create for yourself mentally. Relish (enjoy greatly) these feelings as you take yourself through this journey of excellence.

Is the flame of desire starting to burn yet? It should be!

Part Two—Adversity. The final part of this exercise is optional, for those who believe it can help them based on the guideline below.

When reviewing and/or visualizing your goals, you may also have thought of obstacles that stand in your path toward these goals—perhaps people have told you, or expressed in some manner, their belief that you cannot possibly accomplish what you want. Or maybe there are other types of situations that might present a difficult hurdle for you to overcome before you can achieve your goals.

Whether this exercise will help you or not depends on how thinking about these obstacles makes you feel. If thinking about these people or obstacles starts to deflate your confidence or get you down, then don't use this approach. Stick with the visualization steps in part one above to build on your desire. Visualization *all by itself* is a very powerful means of creating the desire and will to succeed at virtually anything.

However, if thinking about the people and/or obstacles that stand in your way really stings and makes you angry; if it makes you want more than anything to go out and prove to those who doubted you that they were wrong, then go ahead and use these thoughts as a secondary visualization activity. You may find that your level of desire increases dramatically.

As an athlete, the doubt and opposition that I encountered when I told others about my goals made me burn inside and strengthened my resolve into a flaming desire and drive to succeed. You can use this type of internal motivation to increase your level of desire each time you think about it. More adversity just adds more fuel.

If you are one of those rare few who don't have serious obstacles or opposition to your goals, then you can create for yourself the perception or idea of adversity or some sort of adverse situation that puts into question your ability. Then you can use this to fuel your desire to succeed. The example used earlier in this chapter was for a figure skater, gymnast, or diver to perceive the judges as adversaries, since they are the ones who ultimately decide who wins or loses and can take away or give you what you want. But realize, if you do this, that you should only use it to spur you on to success, not as an excuse to fail or a reason to continually talk down or disparage judges.

Chapter 4

Five Letters That Spell Success

The CDSPH Principle—
What It Really Means

COMMITMENT, DISCIPLINE, SACRIFICE, PRIORI-
TIES, HEART—I'll bet you've heard these words many times
before. They are very common in the world of competitive sports.
However, many people throw these terms around without any true
comprehension of them. I hope to get their real meaning across to
you, explain the strong relationship these five qualities have to each
other, and through this process, motivate you toward applying them
to your athletic life. They are crucial in determining the degree to
which you will succeed. For convenience, I have named this group
of intrinsic qualities the CDSPH principle.

In chapter 3, I discussed the importance of desire in attaining
your goals as well as desire's close relationship to passion and motivation. Now, with the help of COMMITMENT, DISCIPLINE,
SACRIFICE, PRIORITIES, and HEART, your passion and motivation become a functional part of accomplishing what you want.

It is one thing to say that you can apply these five concepts, but
it is quite another to actually go out and do it. True champions understand the difference very well and demonstrate their understanding through action. They not only "talk the talk," but they "walk
the walk."

To gain a good grasp of the meaning of these five qualities and
their importance to your success, you must understand what they
mean individually and how they all work together. Let's start with
commitment.

COMMITMENT

When you make a *commitment* to do something, it means that you have firmly decided and, through your own determination, intend to do whatever it takes to do that thing—in this case, fulfill your athletic goals. A commitment is a decision to adhere to a course of action. To *be* committed means to honor a pledge or promise made to yourself to do something.

Dedicated conveys a meaning very similar to *committed*. *Dedicated* means "decided upon, and loyal to, a particular course of thought or action."

As you can see, these two concepts go together. Those who are committed are dedicated and loyal to their goals and often feel passion and other strong emotions like enthusiasm and excitement about the thing they are committed to. In this case, you would feel strong enthusiasm and passion about sticking to your athletic goals and achieving them.

Commitment and *dedication* both include the concept of "self-sacrificing devotion." This means that committed athletes devote themselves to fulfilling their goals and *don't allow other wants or desires that are lower on their priority list to come between them and their commitment.*

Commitment is demonstrated through the consistency with which you apply effort to whatever task, concept, objective, or goal you have decided on. This means working on your goals every day and devoting as much daily time as necessary to the effort. To accomplish consistency and dedication, you may need to *force* yourself to honor and be loyal to the commitments you have made. This, of course, takes *discipline*.

DISCIPLINE AND SACRIFICE

The "discipline" we are talking about here does *not* mean "punishment"! Rather, it means consistently holding yourself to the overall course of action and specific schedule of training that you've decided upon. It means holding to your goals even when something else comes up that might look more interesting at the moment. Without discipline, the athlete is at the mercy of his or her wants and desires, no matter how trivial or unimportant they may be, and this will make it very difficult to make steady progress toward athletic goals.

Some people, for various reasons, find it hard to commit to a schedule. Maybe too often they've had to do things on a schedule that they didn't really want to do, or perhaps they have not taken it upon themselves to exercise their own freedom of choice often enough and therefore haven't had the chance to see what it's like to form their own goals and work toward them. Or perhaps holding to a schedule simply makes them feel like they don't have enough freedom. Whatever the reason, if your desire to excel in athletics is strong enough, and if you realize that this is your own show and it's up to *you* to make it happen (sound familiar?), you can use your logic and intention to decide that it will be worth pursuing despite any sacrifices you have to make.

This is where *sacrifice* comes in. It is during this whole process of disciplining yourself to follow through with your commitment that *sacrifices* are made. When, because of their commitment, athletes do not take part in social activities or behave in a manner that they otherwise might have, they have made a sacrifice. As you progress toward your goals, you will have to do this more often than you might expect. You might have to miss seeing a boyfriend or girlfriend, miss attending a dance or party, skip joining in with something your friends want to do, or whatever. The point is that there will *always* be something that can get in the way of what you, as an athlete, want to accomplish. Tell yourself that this is one of those times you have to make a sacrifice to be true to your goals. Also, setting *priorities* can help you with this.

PRIORITIES

A *priority* is something that is more important than other things. *Setting priorities* means ranking or ordering a number of tasks or actions so the most important ones come first, and the less important ones

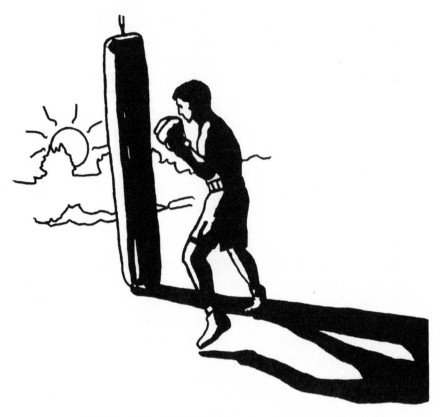

4.1: Disciplined Training Requires Some Sacrifice

follow after those. Assigning priorities to the most important things you are doing is key. Your commitments, including your athletic goals, should be at the top of your priority list, which means that they should be given the highest importance. Setting priorities not only puts what is most important first, but also places importance in *other* aspects of your life—therefore, priorities also help you develop some balance in your life. You should decide what things are important to you and in what order they come.

Be careful though—a dedicated and committed athlete can easily fall prey to an attitude of "all work and no play." On some occasions it is more important to get away from the gym so you can take your mind off all the work and recharge your batteries. When an athlete's training becomes consistently poor over an extended period of time, or if minor aches and pains do not seem to go away, it might be time to take a break.

This situation did not happen to me often during my own training, but it did occur occasionally. What was most amazing was that, more times than not, I showed a noticeable improvement when I came back, as long as the break I took was no more than two or three days. This improvement was not only a physical one, but a mental one as well. I felt both physically and mentally refreshed. This is why keeping a good balance between work and play not only allows for the development of a well-rounded athlete, but can also increase skill performance and training satisfaction.

Just be sure to always honor your commitments first, before anything else—and that includes your commitment toward realizing your athletic goals.

I need to make one more important point before we move forward. This two- or three-day break period I discuss above did include the normal weekly rest day I gave myself, usually Sunday. So during my hard training sessions before the actual season, I might have taken a consecutive Friday, Saturday, and Sunday off, or more likely a Saturday and Sunday, for rest. Again, I normally only took this type of break once or twice, if at all, during my preseason training. Don't confuse this type of break with the longer rest period you might take in order to recuperate mentally and physically after a season (or to play another sport). Even though the short and the long breaks are similar in purpose, the longer rest period has much more importance after a long, hard season.

HEART

The last component of the CDSPH principle is *heart*. I have saved this one for last because it not only helps you to accomplish the first four (especially when doing so is extremely difficult), but it is also the major factor that enables you to create successes in the competitive arena in very intense, difficult situations where everything is at stake. That should sound very familiar because it is eerily similar to what we discussed about *desire* in chapter 3. They do, in fact, come from the same place—inside you.

People can mean somewhat different things when they say that someone has "heart." The most common meaning is "that ephemeral quality an athlete demonstrates when he or she shows such a strong will to succeed or excel that they seem to pull extra ability and hidden reserves of energy and perseverance out of thin air—to somehow keep going, and to go better and faster than everyone else, despite exhaustion, pain, handicaps, or other apparently insurmountable barriers, to achieve the goal."

Therefore, I like to say that heart can be described as the sum of your passion and determination—or, looking at it another way, heart is the ultimate expression of passion and determination. By feeling passion about and exercising determination in your sport, you develop a strong sense of perseverance that can get you through the toughest of times and most competitive of situations—that's heart! Whether you are on your last set of repetitions of a skill while training and you just aren't sure you can finish; whether you are running the final play of a football game and winning or losing is in your hands; or whether you are the last competitor in an event and you know before you go that it will take the best performance of your life to win—all of these take tremendous heart.

The more often the athlete faces these kinds of obstacles and survives, the more heart he or she develops. True champions have deep, strong reserves of heart that they tap into when faced with the most difficult situations. You will be amazed at what you can accomplish with just a little bit of heart. The true champion is a living example of this attribute.

THE MAGIC OF THE CDSPH PRINCIPLE

I would not be doing justice to the CDSPH principle if I did not give one more illustration of the seemingly magic results that can be achieved through holding strong to what this concept implies—in this case, an athlete's skill development. There were times during some of my practice sessions when nothing was going well and it didn't seem as if I would be able to accomplish my daily training objective within a reasonable amount of time. You may have had similar experiences.

What I did in situations like this was discipline myself to simply *finish* the number of repetitions I had committed myself to, even if I had to accept a lower level (quality) of execution. I basically pushed myself through the priorities I had set for my workout. You might think that nothing would be gained by doing this—yet my training the following day was almost always better. It was as if my body had learned or improved from my pushing through the workout, even though I did not subjectively *feel* like I had done anything worthwhile that day.

I have also observed this same phenomenon when teaching new skills to students in physical education. As long as the students force themselves through the difficult motor patterns, even though their movements may not have looked any better, improvement occurred and was noticeable the next day. Basically, the motor skill became easier for them to accomplish. If I had been unable to *discipline* myself through those tough days during my own gymnastic training, I may never have made the steady improvement that I did make—and I may never have picked up on this concept and realized its benefits. So keep this concept in mind in your own training. It could help spell the difference between what you do accomplish and what you don't.

In fact, take a moment to reflect on the earlier stories about Bethany Hamilton, Jim Abbott, Jim MacLaren, and Wilma Rudolph and what they accomplished. What are your thoughts on how committed and disciplined each of them must have been? How about their level of sacrifice, ability to set proper priorities, and amount of heart? Do you think that they just "talked the talk," or did they "walk the walk"?

These champions stand among many other greats who innately *understood* the CDSPH principle and lived it. Take John Wooden.

A GREAT EXAMPLE OF SOMEONE WHO PRACTICED THE CDSPH PRINCIPLE: JOHN WOODEN

One person who personally exemplified, and practiced, the idea of developing the athlete from within was John Wooden. As head basketball coach at the University of California Los Angeles (UCLA) from 1948 through 1975, he accomplished what no college basketball coach had ever done before him, or has since done to date, by winning ten collegiate Division I National Championships, seven of which were consecutive. While coach, his team, the Bruins, "won 81% of their games and set all-time records with four perfect 30–0 seasons, 88 consecutive victories, 38 straight NCAA tournament victories, [and] 20 PAC-10 championships."[1] At this writing, he was one of only three individuals ever inducted into the Naismith Memorial Basketball Hall of Fame both as a player *and* as a coach.[2]

The simple statement by John Wooden's coauthor, Steve Jamison, in the preface of their book, *My Personal Best: Life Lessons from an All-American Journey*, sums it up concisely: "[S]imply, he's an American icon hailed as 'The Greatest Coach of the 20th Century' . . . [who was] awarded the Presidential Medal of Freedom at the White House." In the same preface, Jamison also quoted acclaimed sportswriter Rick Reilly: "There has never been a finer coach in American sports than John Wooden. Nor a finer man."[3]

I wholeheartedly agree. Wooden's ideas were developed over a lifetime of experience as an athlete and coach, with the foundation for many of his principles coming from his strong, traditional family upbringing. I have yet to come across anyone, anywhere, who had a better grasp on what being a true champion is all about. Coach Wooden taught that developing intrinsic values and developing the athlete from within are of huge importance. His belief system centered on what he called "The Pyramid of Success," and it was loaded with intrinsic principles such as industriousness, cooperation, enthusiasm, self-control, confidence, and poise, among others. These are further tied together by other intrinsic concepts, such as honesty, sincerity, integrity, and resourcefulness. All of these qualities build, one upon the other, helping athletes and players reach what Coach Wooden called "competitive greatness" and "success" at the top of his pyramid.[4]

To Coach Wooden, winning games, rather than being the goal or objective, was a *product* and an *outcome* of being and doing your best—in other words, something that happened because of hard work—all things inherent in the CDSPH principle. His goal was to have every athlete under his direction be the very best that they could be. And *that* was the ultimate goal—not whether they won or lost. And, as a result of this emphasis, he and his teams were consistent winners.[5]

I believe that the most important aspect of Coach Wooden's belief system is the fact that it extends well beyond the basketball court and teaches athletes a lot about success in life. There are many players who have competed under his direction who will attest to that fact. Former UCLA Bruin and NBA star Bill Walton put John Wooden's life into fitting perspective:

> John Wooden represents the conquest of substance over hype, the triumph of achievement over erratic flailing, the conquest of discipline over gambling, and the triumph of executing an organized plan over hoping that you'll be lucky, hot or in the zone. John Wooden also represents the conquest of sacrifice, hard work and commitment to achievement over the pipe dream that someone will just give you something, or that you can take a pill or turn a key to get what you want.[6]

If you have not had the opportunity to read any of John Wooden's books or see any of his videotapes or interviews explaining his belief system and its relationship to athletes and success, I strongly urge you to do so.

TAKING ACTION

Picturing the CDSPH Principle

1. To develop a clear picture of what the CDSPH principle might mean to you and give some substance to the definitions I have discussed in this chapter, I would like you to think of things you feel you are committed to and write them down. Try to think of things that you attempt to set aside time for, aim to do on a consistent basis, or hold in very high regard. A simple, unrelated example might just be brushing your teeth. Some people just

don't ever miss their two or three times a day, no matter what, because of concern over good dental hygiene. More relevant examples would include anything you really love to do, want to be good at, or care a great deal about. Write down as many things as you can that you feel might fit into this category of commitments. Any kind of commitment is fine.

2. Now take a good look at your list and cross off any that you do not have a true passion for, or are unable to dedicate consistent time to, or cannot force yourself to "stick with" when things get tough, or are incapable of giving enough priority to. Basically, the things left on your list now come first, very little or nothing gets in your way of doing them, and no matter what, you feel a genuine need to honor them. What you now have on that piece of paper in front of you are your true commitments—the ones you will be able to apply the rest of the CDSPH principle to.

As an athlete, your sport and the training for that sport should be on your list (along with your family and your school work). If they aren't, you will need to take some time to reevaluate the goals you have set for yourself.

· Chapter 5 ·

What You Do Speaks Volumes

Character and Integrity—
The Road Less Traveled

*W*hen you think of the terms *character* and *integrity*, what do you think of? What comes to mind first? Can you think of people who would represent good examples of these terms? How about *not-so-good* examples? Keep these things in mind as we continue through this chapter. It will all become very clear to you shortly.

It has been my observation that character and integrity are important factors in achieving championship form and enduring athletic success. Now, you do see highly skilled and successful athletes in competition who are apparently lacking in either or both of these qualities. This appears to contradict this contention. But I must add that any athlete whose attitude and behavior on *or* off the playing field demonstrate the absence of these two attributes (no matter how successful he or she is) is taking a serious personal risk. Such behavior is not representative of the behavior and standing of a true champion.

Since the importance of character and integrity cannot be underestimated, let's make sure we are both on the same page with regard to their meaning.

CHARACTER AND INTEGRITY

Character. While the word *character* has several related meanings, the one we are using in this chapter is "moral excellence and firmness" (*Merriam-Webster*).[1]

Here is an example of the word *character* used in a sentence:

Her refusal to cheat showed character.

Integrity. *Integrity* is defined by *Oxford American* as "the quality of being honest and having strong moral principles."[2] A synonym of the word *integrity* is *honesty*.

Here is an example of the word *integrity* used in a sentence:

People knew they could trust and rely on Dan because his personal integrity was high.

When we add up what it means to have both character and integrity and look at what kinds of actions are examples of these qualities, we can say that when an athlete possesses good character and integrity, he or she is able to:

- do what is right, good, and just, even though others are not;
- make decisions based on a code of ethical standards that supports the right thing to do, even when no one else is watching;
- stand up for his or her beliefs and principles, even in the face of extreme peer pressure; and
- be honest about mistakes he or she made in situations where character and integrity just weren't great enough to prevent him or her from making them. No one is perfect, and even people possessing the highest level of character make mistakes. Yet their sense of integrity just doesn't allow them to lie about it. Instead, they face up to their mistakes and resolve to do their best to not make them in the future.

CHARACTER AND INTEGRITY
IN ATHLETICS TODAY

It seems to be widely understood and agreed in our society that good character and integrity are attributes that should be revealed and strengthened through participation in athletics. Yet character and integrity, as defined above, often seem to be missing in today's athletes—and many appear to consider them inapplicable. It is just about impossible to pick up a local or national newspaper and not read about an athlete, from high school to professional, who has engaged in behavior and actions completely contrary to the principles mentioned above. You see stories detailing illegal and illicit activities such as drinking, drug use, assaults, hazing, and other unacceptable conduct.

As a teacher, I rarely go through a school year in which no student athletes have been caught participating in such activities. To the contrary, those I did hear about were few compared to the actual number of students engaging in these types of harmful behavior—the ones I knew about represent only the ones who were caught. I would guess that you can attest to this fact based on your own knowledge of what is going on with athletes today, correct?

It is even worse when you consider the professional ranks. Take the use of steroids just as one example. Their covert use became popular at the professional and Olympic levels as a way for athletes to gain an edge on the competition, and their use in professional baseball has only come to the public's attention within recent years. The problem with them is that these drugs give athletes an *unfair* advantage over honest competitors who rely on their own athletic ability and hard work to excel. But unfortunately, the attitude that it's all right to use such shortcuts to physical strength and ability has become pervasive and has filtered down through college sports and even into high school athletics (as have other unethical practices). No matter how you look at it, using drugs to artificially enhance your athletic abilities constitutes cheating, is unhealthful, and is about as far from good character and integrity as you can get.

Unfortunately, there are no real codes of conduct for athletes at the professional level other than the intrinsic values that athletes are supposed to believe in and those that society accepts. This speaks volumes about the state of affairs regarding character and integrity at the highest levels of competition—in other words, it says, loud and clear, that fewer and fewer professional athletes, or their organizations, place a high value on character and integrity. This is reflected in the frequent news stories about professional athletes suspended from teams or arrested for drug and steroid use, sexual misconduct, and other illegal and unethical activities (we will discuss these issues further in chapter 6, "An Unrewarding Path").

ATHLETIC CODES

Athletic codes are normally set up by a school system for the purpose of supporting and developing the character and integrity of its athletes. The student athlete's signature on the code is intended to be a promise to honor and abide by the principles set out within the code. The majority of precepts in these codes center on the idea that an athlete needs to set sound ethical and moral examples for others to aspire to and should *not* exhibit behavior and participate in activities that are illegal, forbidden, unbecoming of a person in such a position, or which inhibit the development and success of the team, or teams, for which they play. These are sound principles that are intended to help formulate good character and integrity, and the athlete (*you*) should feel obligated and honored to uphold them. Athletes' signatures should be their word, and their word should be their firm promise. Yet adherence to the athletic codes athletes have signed appears to be more of a fantasy than a reality.

Case in point, a number of years ago there was a high school student athlete who decided to chronicle his weekend activities on videotape during his senior year. His purpose, I would guess, was to create a memento of his last year in high school. So he took his video camera along to the various parties he attended and recorded the many goings-on at these "social gatherings," whatever their nature.

As luck would have it, he had a project coming due for one of the classes he was taking, and video was the medium he used. But he inadvertently recorded the assignment on the same videotape he had been using to chronicle his senior year activities. He then turned his project in to his teacher, unknowingly including everything else that was on the tape.

To say that his recordings caused an uproar would be a serious understatement. The teacher was floored by what she saw and promptly turned the tape in to the athletic department. Consumption of alcohol, signs of other drug use, sexually tinged behavior—all were there for the viewing.

Coaches of the various sports at the school were called in to identify athletes on their teams, and many were in shock and disbelief at the sheer number of athletes on the tape, who they were, and the types of behavior these athletes exhibited.

Regrettably, violations of athletic codes are commonplace at the high school level. The proof of this lies in the answer to the following question: How many student athletes do you know who consistently follow their own school's athletic codes? My experience as a coach, teacher, athlete, and parent has shown me that there are not enough who do. In fact, many parents and athletes sign these codes without really giving much thought to them or even reading them. They are just thought of as part of the process they have to go through in order to play their sport.

Additionally, for those aware of what their athletic code covers, learning, understanding, and abiding by it can be very difficult if others turn a blind eye to, condone, or even support activities that break it. Some athletes and their parents tend to look at these codes as "unfair" because the school "forces" the athlete to sign them in order to play. Student athletes have been known to try to skirt the rules and consequences that occur when they are caught in violation. They have taken their cases to court, made excuses, and even lied in order to keep themselves on the playing field.

The problem is that these attitudes create an environment where it becomes nearly impossible for athletes to develop good character and integrity. Competitors learn from the poor examples set by others that "the rules" do not apply to them. This tears a gaping hole in the fabric of these two moral and ethical principles by demonstrating that neither character nor integrity really matters. So, rather than helping to support the idea of taking responsibility for their own actions when athletes stray off the path of honesty or good behavior, the environment—friends, team members, parents, the behavior of professional athletes, and others—in effect tells them that they can get away with bad or, in some cases, illegal and destructive actions and not have to suffer any consequences.

I want you to think about that for a moment. Do you believe this to be the type of lesson athletes like yourself should learn? Do you think it might possibly have any far-reaching consequences for athletes later, when they go out on their own in the real world? Athletes need to recognize and understand that the code is a means by which schools set parameters for the development of good, sound, lifelong values. You need to recognize and understand this fact.

Even though this discussion focuses attention primarily on high school athletic codes, most colleges also have similar forms of athletic codes of conduct. College athletic codes, like their high school counterparts, promote positive behavior and good sportsmanship while discouraging athletes from engaging in any form of illegal, illicit, or unethical behavior. They are meant to encourage the development of good character and integrity. Despite such college codes of conduct, however, poor and destructive behavior is far too common among college athletes. A Google search of "college athletes behaving badly" brings up numerous hits, among them a website called badjocks.com. This website is dedicated to exposing the poor character choices of anyone involved in sports, including college athletes.

Why am I making such a fuss over character and integrity? *Because they form a significant part of the foundation for anything and everything that an athlete is trying to accomplish!* They help to support and intensify the CDSPH principle (discussed in chapter 4) through the development of inner strength and a strong work ethic. Most important, they transcend sports by going beyond the athletic arena and becoming a road map by which athletes can live their lives—by which *you* can live *your* life.

Good character and integrity are not necessarily something you are born with, but they are values that you can develop when you make the right choices. These two attributes should be part of the core principles every individual seeks to develop. They are something to aspire to, and something to be proud of. It is my firm opinion that no matter how successful an athlete becomes, the amount of character and integrity he or she demonstrates is what separates the true champion from all others.

When athletes habitually disregard the common precepts of moral and ethical behavior that civilized society around them adheres to, it is very easy to engage in cheating. In the next chapter, we take up cheating in its various forms, its prevalence, and what the harmful downside to cheating consists of.

TAKING ACTION

Making the Right Choice

Using an example of an athletic code from high school, let's take a look at how you might apply the information covered in this chapter so far. Most athletic codes expect athletes to stay away from the use of drugs and tobacco and the consumption of alcohol—activities that are illegal for most kids of high school age. Some codes even take this a step further by considering that even an athlete's mere presence at a location (like a party) where these activities are being engaged in by teens is a violation of the code, whether or not the athlete himself or herself is using or consuming.

Using the above "mere presence" athletic code precept for our hypothetical situation, assume that a male athlete who has signed this code walks into a party where his friends and peers are drinking and using drugs. All his friends are there, they all seem to be having a good time, and what are the chances that he will get caught, right? Based on our discussion in this chapter, what should he do? What choice should he make that would demonstrate good character and integrity? What would you do? Do the answers you give for this athlete and for yourself represent the concepts covered in this chapter?

There is no argument about how tough this kind of situation might be for you or for anyone in this situation and, in all likelihood, you will find yourself in a similar situation at some point. However, isn't that what demonstrating strong character and integrity is all about? Tough choice, yes, but is there really any other option for you than to walk out that door, if you want to apply what you've learned in this chapter?

We could take this even further by assuming the athlete stays, gets caught, and his parents and/or coach find out about this violation. Now everyone involved, including the adults, will be putting their character and integrity on the line. What will the parents do? Will they support the integrity of the code they, too, signed and hold their child accountable? Or will they fight the school so their kid can still play? What will the coach do? If the athlete caught in violation is considered a "star" and is needed on the field of play for the team to win, will the coach put winning above all else, or will he or she teach the proper lesson? I am sure you would be able to tell both parties what the *right* thing to do would be.

· Chapter 6 ·

An Unrewarding Path

Cheating—The Road to Nowhere

$\mathcal{A}$s I detail for you how cheating has become more commonplace in the sports world, I want you to think about its relevance to one's character and integrity—*your* character and integrity—and why some athletes feel the need to stoop to such a level.

At first glance it should seem obvious that cheating and the qualities of a "true champion" would not coexist in the same person. However, this may not be so easy to see when you look at current sports at all levels of competition. Many of our so-called sports heroes, despite their athletic attainments, don't fit the mold of a true champion. This is one of the reasons why I personally would have so much difficulty labeling many of them as such, and why we have included a chapter in this book about *cheating*. After all, we are striving toward reaching that goal of true champion.

WHAT IS CHEATING?

First, let's break down the meaning of *cheating* as we are using it here. Any time a competitor tries to seek an *unfair* advantage over the competition, does not follow the rules of the game, and/or engages in drugging that can give them an advantage while being detrimental to their health over the long term, they are cheating. Whether you use performance-enhancing drugs, whether you buddy up to an official to get the call, or whether you deliberately try to hurt your opponent, all these actions seek an unfair advantage—a *shortcut* to success.

But a shortcut to success really has *nothing* to do with success at all. *If you don't follow the rules of the game, you haven't played the game.* Any game consists of play according to certain exact rules. If you are violating or avoiding or cheating on those rules, then you aren't really playing, and any "success" or win you have as a result is a false or phony success—it's not something one can take any real pride in. Someone who cheats has forfeited their character and their integrity.

The above types of cheating fall under the heading of "short-term gratification" (discussed in the introduction and in chapter 1)—a misguided way of looking at athletics and competition that has become pervasive in our society today. Too many athletes, from high school through professional levels, take the attitude that the right objective is "winning at all costs." This attitude has also brought with it the idea that doing something that is not exactly "right" is fine and acceptable *as long as you do not get caught.* I have stood in amazement when, in casual conversations with students and student athletes, they have voiced this belief.

The problem with this attitude is that YOU know you cheated—and how can you respect *yourself* if you cheat? It is really hard—you have to give yourself all kinds of brainless excuses—and then you have to *believe* your dim-witted self! Better to admit you cheated and resolve never to do it again. If you continually deny—even to yourself—that you are doing anything wrong, who do you really think you are fooling? Cheating and its innate self-denial have the consequence of causing your character to start rotting away from the inside out, if you continue.

What occurs is that cheating hurts one's ability to reap the intrinsic rewards that come from hard work and commitment to the achievement of goals. True success in all its dimensions is only experienced when you dedicate yourself to following the "right" path—when you do "what is right." That's right—no matter what you have heard, whether from teachers, counselors, friends, or even parents, there IS a right path to follow and there IS a wrong path—and the wrong path always involves shortcuts or risks that a true champion is *not* willing to take. At its simplest, the "right way" means following all the rules of the game and your school or organization's athletic code of conduct, and not cheating on them.

HOW COMMON HAS CHEATING BECOME?

In the past, the act of cheating brought with it ethical, moral, and, sometimes, legal consequences definitely not associated with a positive athletic experience. There was a clear line between right and wrong, and cheating definitely fell on the wrong side of the tracks. Today, this line appears to have become blurred. What is the reason for this change in attitude?

Let me start by stating that I do not believe that this lax attitude is anything new. There have always been individuals who have wanted to skirt the rules or cheat in order to win or succeed. However, it seems to me that this belief has become more acceptable and is now being viewed as inevitable and thus "OK" by too many in society. I draw this conclusion not only from my experiences as a teacher, but also from the questionable role models many athletes are trying to emulate.

As an example, take a look at the revelations and controversy regarding the use of performance-enhancing drugs in a professional sport such as major league baseball (MLB). As documented in the video of a press conference given by former MLB outfielder Jose Canseco on May 7, 2009, discussing the charges of widespread steroid use in major league baseball revealed in his book *Juiced*, released in February 2005, Canseco alleged "that [steroid use] was as wild and as rampant as maybe 80 to 90% of the players."[1] Canseco's charges have been disputed by players and other figures in major league baseball, some even stating that he made them just so he could sell lots of copies of his book.

Let's just say, for the sake of argument, that Canseco's 80 percent figure was exaggerated, even two or three times. Whether you accept Canseco's perspective verbatim, other current players' perspectives, or a combination of both, you still have to conclude that there is definitely a lot of cheating occurring. These players are seeking an *unfair* advantage over others—cheating—with the underlying objective likely being to "win," as well as fame, money, and the other benefits (some legal and others not) that are easily available to top sports figures.

In order to shed more light on how deeply into pro baseball this type of cheating has spread, let me take you through some recent past events in this century's worst steroid scandal. In April 2006, major league baseball commissioner Bud Selig announced that the issue of steroid use in major league baseball would be addressed. He appointed former U.S. senator George Mitchell to head a panel to investigate allegations leveled against major league ballplayers regarding their use of performance-enhancing drugs. The inquiry was set to investigate, among others, renowned home-run hitter, San Francisco Giants' Barry Bonds, against whom serious drugging allegations had been raised.[2]

On May 28, 2006, Bonds became the first player to exceed Babe Ruth's home-run record, hitting his 715th career home run. Then on August 7, 2007, Bonds hit his 756th home run, breaking the all-time career home-run record formerly held by Hank Aaron. The sheer immensity of these accomplishments, when considered in light of the allegations and, at the date of this writing, the probability of Bonds's steroid use, cast an even darker shadow over these achievements and increased the possibility that many other purportedly stellar records in this and other sports would be invalidated.

Mr. Mitchell's report went public on December 13, 2007, and it probed much more deeply into what it called the "steroid era" than just the allegations against Bonds. During the investigation, over seven hundred witnesses were interviewed, 550 of whom were current/former club officials, managers, team physicians, coaches, athletic trainers, and resident security agents. Actual evidence of drug deals and purchases in the form of numerous telephone records, receipts, and other types of documents were documented. The report concluded that steroids and performance-enhancing substances had been used by players in major league baseball at all levels for over ten years. This included players who may someday be considered for the Baseball Hall of Fame. Even though Jose Canseco's claim of 80 percent player drug usage was not necessarily supported, and a variety of different percentages were indicated by other players (none of which can be verified), the report did state:

> [T]he evidence we uncovered indicates that this has not been an isolated problem involving just a few players or a few clubs. It has involved many players on [sic] many clubs. In fact, each of the thirty clubs has had players who have been involved with performance-enhancing substances at some time in their careers.

Evidence in the Mitchell report substantiated the pervasive use of steroids and human growth hormone in major league baseball for "all" levels of players. It also made reference, however brief, to the fact that this problem is not exclusive to baseball (discussed immediately below).[3]

Even though the use of these substances is illegal and illicit, unfair, and a form of cheating; even though it forwards the erroneous goal of "winning at all costs" and can have serious physical, emotional, and mental consequences, my biggest issue with performance-enhancing drug and steroid use is the unethical example major league ballplayers are setting for aspiring athletes like you. It speaks loud and clear as to the poor character and integrity of the players who use these substances, and it destroys any possibility, for any athlete engaging in this behavior, for the development of the intrinsic values indicative of a true champion.

As mentioned above, athletes in other professional sports have also been implicated in the use of illegal performance-enhancing drugs. The 2007 suspension and eventual confession of professional cyclist Floyd Landis of having used performance-enhancing drugs "for most of his career as a professional road cyclist,"[4] and the suspension and admission of NFL linebacker Brian Cushing in 2010 for violating the NFL's anti-doping policy by taking a banned performance-enhancing substance, are examples.[5] Even seven-time Tour de France champion Lance Armstrong (a former teammate of Floyd Landis), as of 2011, was under investigation in the face of ongoing allegations of performance-enhancing drug use.[6]

Moreover, Olympic-level sports have not escaped the allure and use of these substances and practices. Track and field is a prime example, rampant with allegations and suspensions. An article posted on July 17, 2004, at USAToday.com reported that Regina Jacobs had been suspended by the U.S. Anti-Doping Agency (USADA) for four years after she tested positive for a known steroid, THG. This athlete had won twelve national titles in the 1,500 meter dash, but had to forfeit her twelfth championship. What was most interesting and bothersome about the article was not only Ms. Jacobs's involvement and suspension but the number of other Olympic- and national-caliber athletes it reported had been named as having also tested positive for performance-enhancing substances, including world-class sprinter, Tim Montgomery, the world-record holder in the 100 meter.[7] In 2005, the USADA formally announced charges against Tim Montgomery for alleged steroid use. Montgomery was barred for two years from track and field by the Court of Arbitration for Sport, and his activities were linked to the investigation of BALCO, the lab that was alleged to have provided steroids to a number of sports figures. Then in April 2007, the extent of Montgomery's illegal activities became clear as he pleaded guilty to conspiracy in a multimillion-dollar bank fraud and money-laundering scheme and was sentenced to nearly four years in prison.[8] He was also convicted and sentenced to five years in prison in 2008 for dealing heroin.[9]

As you can see, this doping and illegal activity was occurring at the very top of the sport. On October 5, 2007, champion sprinter Marion Jones, the winner of three gold medals and two bronzes in various track and field events at the 2000 Sydney Summer Olympics (and former girlfriend of Tim Montgomery), tearfully admitted to lying to federal investigators, and to steroid use beginning in 1999 while training for the 2000 Summer Olympics. She was suspended from competition for two years and was stripped of the three gold and two bronze medals she won in Sydney. Her track and field career was over: she retired the same day.[10]

If I were to include the full list of alleged, convicted, and/or suspended national and Olympic track athletes involved in the use of these drugs, it would be quite long.

After all the negative publicity, suspensions, and other consequences doled out to past and current athletes who made the poor choice to cheat through the use of performance-enhancing substances, you would think that the 2008 Beijing Summer Olympics might have represented a turning point toward more positive behavior—but you would be wrong. An Internet search of "steroids in the Beijing Olympics" turned up many hits. With athletes from a variety of sports and countries suspended for positive tests even before the games began, and at least six disqualified during the games, the hope of "clean" competitions at the Olympics, or at any elite level, for that matter, seemed more like a pipe dream than a possibility. It is no wonder that so many of us now question every record-breaking performance. We wonder, "Are they using, or aren't they?"

Athletes who cheat may also believe, mistakenly, that use of performance-enhancing drugs is the only way to become the "best" and that use of these drugs is the only way to keep up with the competition.

But remember:

Athletic achievement attained through the unfair advantage of performance-enhancing drugs is simply not real achievement.

If enough people use steroids, athletics becomes not a game of individual ability, but of who can use the "best" drugs to artificially build up their athletic ability the most. By doing this, an athlete has left the arena of honest sports competition far behind and is instead engaging in a competition of chemicals and chemical effects. The bottom line must be that cheating is still cheating. Eventually there *will* be a negative consequence to these athletes, be it internal or external, no matter if the cheater is caught or not.

The lure of winning at all costs, as well as the fame and fortune that accompany professional- and elite-level sports celebrity, all fall under the category of *extrinsic* motivators, and these appear to be (directly or indirectly) among the primary motivations for illegal performance-enhancement practices among our top-level athletes. These extrinsic motivations are not something I personally could ever associate with a true champion. As is almost always the case, when outside factors are an athlete's primary objective rather than the intrinsic benefits of doing well in the sport, trouble follows, with character and integrity being the sacrifice. Yet, these outside influences (fame, fortune, winning at all costs) seem to increasingly lie behind the rise in cheating in many sports.

A very serious result of this type of cheating is not only that it involves the destruction of the athlete's intrinsic benefits and rewards—the benefits I am encouraging you to seek—but also that it destroys their integrity. How can any of these athletes really respect themselves after doing this? I mean, how can anyone really take pride in an "accomplishment" or win that occurred as a result of an advantage obtained through drug use? It is obvious that these athletes have become so obsessed with the mere end result or *appearance* of winning—winning at all costs—that they have forgotten what "winning" really means. Sadly, many athletes who cheat with drugs still work very hard in their sports! If they only realized how they were wasting all that hard work by polluting their accomplishments with chemical assistance. Why not gain a clean victory and know that the final result of your hard work was clearly and, without any doubt whatsoever, solely due to your own dedicated effort?

PHYSICAL CONSEQUENCES OF CHEATING WITH PERFORMANCE-ENHANCING DRUGS

Completely aside from the loss of integrity entailed by cheating with performance-enhancing drugs, there is the question of the negative short- and long-term side effects that can result from the use of these chemicals. Laboratory and human studies have shown that steroid use is associated with many harmful changes in organs and systems of the body. The best-documented negative effects are those on the liver, blood composition, and the reproductive system, but steroid use carries the risk of many other serious side effects.

Potential harmful effects on males include decrease in male hormones, testicle size, sperm count, sperm motility, and increases in tendon injuries. Likewise, potential effects on women include menstrual abnormalities, deeper voice, decrease in breast size, balding, acne, body hair, and increase in clitoral size. Moreover, these above effects don't begin to detail the possible negative psychological and behavioral changes, most notably in males. These dangers are discussed in a March 2005 article in the *Research Digest* of the President's Council on Physical Fitness and Sports coauthored by Dr. Charles E. Yesalis, one of the foremost U.S. experts on the nonmedical use and abuse of anabolic-androgenic steroids (AS) and performance-enhancing drugs, and Dr. Michael S. Bahrke, an expert in exercise physiology and sports psychology.[11]

Additionally, other possible negative side effects and health complications may exist but not yet be known, as only time and years of research can give us the answers to that question.

So what is to be gained by the use of these substances? For the true champion, not a thing, for he or she will understand that their use is a form of cheating. True champions are what they are because of the inner rewards they realize through their efforts rather than the status of winning and being a "superstar" or the money and other material benefits that may accompany the accomplishment of their goals. True champions are interested in real achievement, not in the *pretense of achievement* by the use of performance-enhancing drugs to gain these material and monetary rewards.

THE "OTHER" KIND OF CHEATING

What about the "other" type of cheating going on in professional sports, which has been most publicized in the NBA? I'm not talking about the kind of cheating that wins games unfairly, but the kind that can destroy a marriage. An example was Kobe Bryant's widely reported encounter and alleged sexual assault of a woman in 2004, and before that, the paternity suit filed against Michael Jordan in 2002. Kobe's charges were dismissed; however, he did not deny he had had sexual relations with the woman.[12] Two negative DNA tests cleared Jordan of the paternity charge,[13] but the disagreement was not over whether he had engaged in extramarital affairs, but whether he was the father of the woman's child. No matter what the detailed facts were in either case, there is no argument that both athletes did cheat on their wives.

Even though this discussion focuses on the NBA, basketball is far from the only professional sports environment where this type of behavior is taking place. It is pretty well known in the sporting world that a good number of professional "superstar" athletes in all sports engage in promiscuity and adultery—marriage notwithstanding.

One of the biggest stories to ever hit the mass media on this issue broke in late 2009 about superstar golfer Tiger Woods. Formerly a strong contender for what I have defined as a true champion, Woods broke all rules of good character and integrity by engaging in numerous extramarital affairs. After the first story of his adultery went public, so many women came forward with similar allegations that it was difficult to keep track of them all! It appeared that Tiger's appetite for promiscuous affairs had been at a level equal to his aspirations of winning golf tournaments.[14]

At this point, you might be asking yourself how any of *this* type of cheating relates to success in sports. It has become common in the world of athletes (and in the society in general), so what's the problem? Let me answer that question in this manner.

These three individuals (Bryant, Jordan, and Woods) are very highly regarded in their sports—and not only as athletes, but also as people that many others want to emulate—especially aspiring athletes like you. With the bad examples these three have given us, competitors can easily make the mistake of believing that this kind of behavior is supposed to be a *part* of being a successful or famous athlete.

No, it decidedly is *not*. You need to realize that cheating is cheating and it is dishonest. When it occurs, no matter what form it may take, it negatively impacts the person *as a whole* and can negatively influence other areas of their lives, including the types of decisions they make. It hurts their families and others close to them. Face it—someone who cheats on his or her girlfriend, boyfriend, or spouse has no integrity—they are lying to those closest to them. If they become known as someone who lies and can't be trusted, it can result in losing their loved ones—and eventually their friends. Cheating in one area of your life can easily have a detrimental impact in many other areas of your life. A simple look at what happened to Tiger certainly supports this possibility: the loss of endorsements, divorce from his wife, and struggles to regain his earlier golfing form and stature. All are likely fallout from his cheating behavior.

THE END RESULTS OF CHEATING

Cheating of any kind chips away at the foundations of who you are as a person—you know, those positive attributes we have been talking about throughout Section I and that I am strongly encouraging you to adopt. Cheating of any kind diminishes your ability to make sound, rational decisions—the kinds of decisions that allow a person to develop their capabilities as fully as possible and realize their full potential.

One meaning of integrity is "whole"—a person who has integrity is whole as a person: honest in all their relationships with others, and not hiding things from others. On the other hand, it's obvious that someone who is cheating is being dishonest and hiding things from others, pretending to be one thing to some people and another to other people—in other words, splitting themselves into pieces, showing different faces to different people rather than being one whole, honest person whom everyone can trust.

You have to realize that when you cheat, you are also being dishonest with *yourself.* You are lying to yourself, telling yourself that cheating will make you come out on top, or make you feel better, or have the most fun—when, in reality, it can put you at the bottom, busted, maybe even stuck with a serious, debilitating illness, and possibly in jail, with people mistrusting you and not wanting to be around you. The consequences of cheating can amount to a ruined, miserable life.

I know these words may seem harsh and unforgiving when it comes to cheating and its negative impact on one's character and integrity. The whole idea here is to get you to think about the *right* choices before heading down such a path.

All that said, I do not believe that character and/or integrity are absolutes in the sense that, once degraded or lost, they can never be regained. No one is perfect and people, whether athletes or not, do make mistakes. The key, I think, once someone realizes they've made a mistake, is that they have the integrity to admit—especially to themselves—that their choice or choices *were* wrong. They should be able to admit that they recognize *what* was wrong about their actions, and sincerely vow *not* to repeat such behavior. The degree to which their character can be restored and their integrity regained will be determined by their ability to hold steadfastly to this commitment to not repeat those poor choices, and perhaps to strive to be and do better than ever before. Any person willing to turn a situation like that into a positive, not only for themselves but for others too, should be given the respect earned and deserved by such an act.

So what's the best overall course of action? Hold out for being honest, for being worthy of trust, for the inner rewards and satisfaction that doing the right thing will bring you. These rewards are the very best kind—they last your entire life and are one of the foundations of real happiness and fulfillment.

TAKING ACTION
A True Winner

Here's a possible situation with which you can test your ability to apply what we've discussed in this chapter. What if you were taking a class that was very important to you and you wanted to get an A in that class? So, you study really hard and sacrifice time with friends and doing other things you enjoy because of the importance you have placed on accomplishing your goal of getting an A. Then you take the final exam in this class at the end of the semester, and even though you have done everything you can, you receive a B on the exam. This ends up giving you a B+ in the course because of the grading curve used on this test.

After class, on the last day, several of your classmates are talking in the hall, and you overhear how many of them cheated on this final exam and got an A. They all laugh and kid each other about how easy it was for them to do this. However, you know that the fact that these students cheated altered the grading curve and made it much harder on anyone getting a grade lower than the cheating students. Now what comes to your mind first about this situation? How does it make you feel? Did the "right" students get the A's in this class? Was everybody evaluated on an even playing field? Did they really "win" that A?

It's amazing how clear things become when looking at a situation armed with sound principles.

· Chapter 7 ·

A Championship
State of Mind

Core Attitudes and a
Mind-Set for Achievement

It's time for us to head deeper into how you should *think* about training and competition, for it is how you think that will determine what you will actually be able to *do*.

This thinking process centers on your perspective or state of mind. The term I use for this perspective is *mind-set*—it refers to how you think about your athletic endeavors and objectives and how you direct your intentions. The first thing to realize is that you *have* the ability to control your own mind-set. It is not up to any other thing, person, emotion, factor, unexpected occurrence, or position of the planets or full moon—it is simply up to *you*!

PROPER MIND-SET: BELIEF IN YOURSELF

One of the characteristics of a proper mind-set is the belief you have in yourself. We have all heard the cliché "you must believe to achieve." It is actually much more than just a cliché—it is an attitude—and an attitude is a mind-set that you consciously adopt. True belief in yourself brings with it the confidence needed for successful training and greatly increases the possibility that you will eventually accomplish your goals.

For example, take again the stories already presented in this book about Bethany Hamilton, Jim MacLaren, Jim Abbott, and Wilma Rudolph. All four labored through tremendous adversity. What do you think their attitudes about themselves were—their belief in themselves? Do you think they would have accomplished what they did without a very strong conviction that they could succeed at what they wanted to do? What was it that made them not give up in the face of such difficulty? I am sure you know the answer. I know Anthony Robles does.

Who is Anthony Robles? Anthony was the wrestler from Arizona State who defeated the defending national champion in the 125-pound weight division to win the NCAA Division I National Championship in 2011.[1] This achievement alone is enough to support how important believing in yourself is to one's success. However, there is something else—something I have purposefully left out of the story. It is a piece that undoubtedly brings more relevance to that cliché, "you must believe to achieve." You see, Anthony, our champion wrestler, was born with only *one leg*. That is correct; he wrestled and defeated an able-bodied wrestler, the defending national champion, on one of the biggest stages in wrestling, and he did it as a one-legged athlete. This does not happen without the belief that *you can*!

Belief in yourself comes from deep within your gut. It starts, like so many other principles, with a choice and a decision—the choice and decision that you *can* do what it takes to accomplish the goals you have set. It starts just like it did with Robles, Hamilton, MacLaren, Abbott, and Rudolph, who *all* chose to believe that they *could* accomplish their goals. Only when you consciously choose this attitude can you build upon it and strengthen it. And your belief in yourself will naturally strengthen as you experience successes during practice and in competition.

You should realize, however, that successes only occur with proper training (something I cover thoroughly in Section II), and proper training only occurs when you bring the right attitude into the gym. This becomes what I refer to as the "circle of success." It is why athletes who succeed tend to keep on succeeding. It begins, as stated several times above, with a conscious choice—the choice that you *can* accomplish your goals. Everything flows from this choice.

CONFIDENCE, NOT ARROGANCE

Keep in mind that true champions don't demonstrate their belief in themselves through arrogance and boasting. Real confidence is demonstrated not through cockiness, but in a much subtler and quieter manner. The famous statement made by President Theodore Roosevelt, "Speak softly and carry a big stick," fits this idea nicely. In fact, it is almost always true that the more any individual feels he or she *has* to repeatedly assert and verbalize how good they think they are (or can be), the less confidence they really have. Self-confidence is internal—something you possess and don't need to broadcast to everyone, whereas arrogance is the pretense of superiority without real possession of it. It is usually pretty easy for others to tell the difference between arrogance and real self-confidence. Remember, however, that there is no need to hide your accomplishments or affect false modesty; there is nothing wrong with self-confidence or the physical poise and self-control that accompany athletic skill. On the contrary, they are part of it.

TAKING CALCULATED RISKS

Another important characteristic that develops through belief in yourself is the ability to take educated or calculated risks. What I mean by "educated" is that the risk itself is thought through and the downside *and* upside are worked out (and all this can be done in the blink of an eye and under extreme pressure by the self-confident athlete). If the athlete takes a calculated risk and is successful, it brings great benefits to the athlete and/or the team.

With the score tied and only seconds left on the clock, John works himself free from the double-team that has been dogging him all game long.

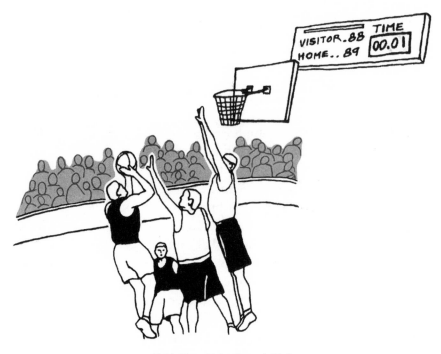

7.1: The Calculated Risk

His teammates are looking for him to get open as he is by far the best and most confident scorer on the team. As John breaks into the open, a teammate passes him the ball, the opponent's defense adjusts quickly, and two defenders rapidly converge on his position. Just as quickly John assesses the situation, and with the game in his hands, and with one second left, he takes the shot . . .

A competitor who understands that he or she can create opportunities through a calculated risk that would not have existed without it is much more willing to take a gamble on such a risk. Whether you want to take that last shot to win or lose the game, or whether you decide to perform the more difficult skill because without it the team may not be successful, does not really matter. What matters is that all of these choices involve the same kind of risk, and the person willing to take that risk will be the athlete who believes he or she can win.

The opposite of this attitude and willingness is to be *un*willing to take such a risk, or to just let someone else do it—usually because of the fear of failure. But champions know that any failure that occurs while taking these risks is temporary and short-term, and that you have the ability to turn them into positive experiences because you will learn from them.

The result of taking calculated risks is that you increase your chances (and motivation) to succeed the next time. To be a successful athlete you must have the confidence to *want* the ball when the game is on the line. Believing in yourself is where that confidence comes from.

And keep in mind that being highly successful with calculated risks, as with everything in this book, is built upon all the foundations we have discussed and will discuss as we venture through the building of a true champion. All are *interconnected*.

RESPONSIBILITY

The next component of a good mind-set is something I highlighted in chapter 1, the *willingness to be responsible*; its importance here should not be taken lightly.

This principle is also part of the belief system that a person chooses, and in fact, responsibility has everything to do with choice. Many people believe that taking responsibility only means "accepting blame for something bad that happened." That's because it is used in that sense so often. But this is not what I'm talking about. "Responsibility" has a much higher meaning. Taking responsibility ultimately means that *you know that you are the one who causes your own success and will act accordingly*. This is one of the most important things I can tell you about excelling in sports.

You are the one who causes your own success.

I detailed for you earlier that responsibility, or rather, the readiness to take on responsibility, is one of the principles that many athletes seem to have a problem with. Many people, young and old, have begun taking the attitude that their success and/or failure is governed largely by others (rather than themselves). They believe that someone "must give us something" in order for us to succeed, and conversely, if they fail, someone or something else must have been to blame.

Society may currently be more accepting of this view than in the past; however, *you cannot afford to be.* At least not if you are seeking to reach levels of performance that your potential dictates you can reach. Keep something very important in mind—when an athlete adopts an attitude that they *cannot* succeed because of someone or something outside of themselves, they automatically give up their responsibility to overcome any obstacle. This is a *losing* attitude. You should never justify failing or losing by looking for excuses and scapegoats and others to blame; there are literally endless reasons that can be dreamed up for an athlete's poor performance or poor standing on a team. What you should be doing is learning from these setbacks and thinking about ways *you* can overcome obstacles in your path.

The further you can distance yourself from this idea of excuse-making and the more responsibility you take on yourself for your own success, the better off you will be. As I said previously, if an athlete is *not* getting something he or she wants or needs in order to be successful (for example, sufficient practice time, or practice of the right skills), it is their responsibility to go out and get it. This cannot be made any simpler! Rather than giving *someone else* power over your success, take the attitude that you are the one who causes your own success. This puts much more control over what happens to you, and for you, into your own hands. That is as it should be. It is what taking responsibility is all about.

Take control over your own destiny by taking responsibility for your own success and for achieving the goals you set for yourself!

KNOWING YOUR STRENGTHS AND WEAKNESSES

Another core attitude of one's mind-set that can enhance your chances of success as an athlete involves knowing your strengths and weaknesses. All competitors have areas or parts of their "game" that are stronger than others. It is important to be honest with yourself about these, because once you are aware of your strengths and weaknesses, a very important philosophy for improvement can be applied:

You will work on developing your weaknesses (weak areas) into strengths, and you will take your strengths (strong areas) to the level of mastery.

Applying this philosophy does two things. First, it forces you to concentrate and work on areas that need the most improvement. This will always increase your ability. Too many athletes spend the majority of their time on areas they are already good at and little if any time on areas they are not good at. Why? Because it is not fun to work on your weakest skills. However, to reach championship levels, competitors must take the time to work on their weaknesses, whether they like doing it or not.

It will be during this process that you will find instances where you are unable to improve on your weaker areas quickly enough, and you *may* have to alter or *adapt* your approach in order to achieve what you want. Sometimes a different technique, strategy, or even perspective on something you're having trouble with can make a big difference in the outcome. There were several occasions in my own career, especially in high school, where I had to make a change of direction in order to achieve my goal or goals, and you'll read about them in Section III. Of course, discovering the need to adapt would never have occurred if I had not spent a good deal of time trying to improve weaker areas. In all likelihood, the same will be true for you. This is another reason why spending time focusing and training in areas you are *not* good at is so important.

The second reason for applying this philosophy of knowing and working on both your strengths and weaknesses is one that cannot be emphasized enough: this approach allows you to take your strengths *beyond* what is considered good execution, up to a very high level of mastery. Working toward this level of accomplishment gives you the freedom to develop your own style and put your unique signature on your work. Perfecting your skills, techniques, and strategies in this manner can be very rewarding, and it will likely place you far above your competition.

Think about that for a moment—how great would it be for you to be known for the uniqueness and style you bring to something you do in your sport? It is a very rewarding *and* humbling experience.

If you are to succeed in these two related endeavors, you must take the time to thoroughly dissect both your strongest and weakest skills into their smaller parts—break them down. This will help you discover what really makes them tick, increasing your ability to enhance both and execute them at their highest level. Once you've done this, it is just a matter of applying the training principles covered throughout this book.

Working on both your strong *and* weak areas can have a tremendously positive impact on your performance.

STRIVING TOWARD PERFECTION

It is important to understand that none of what I have discussed so far, and will continue to discuss, is going to be easy. If it were, everyone would do it. But mediocrity is not acceptable to a champion. Athletes seeking the highest level of achievement for themselves— those who are striving toward perfection—will practice, *with a very high level of focus*, skills, techniques, strategies, plays, or anything else that will improve their performance or enhance their chances of success, and they will practice until they achieve the level of skill acceptable to them. It is not that they *expect* absolute perfection from themselves—but they will *strive for it* as hard as they can, literally pushing themselves to practice their skills at the very edge of their capabilities.

This might seem like a contradiction to some. Why don't champions expect absolute perfection, and why strive for it if they don't expect to really reach it? Well, there are several things to understand about the idea of perfection here, as it relates to sports. First of all, "perfection" by itself isn't anything mysterious. Every time an athlete envisions the right or best way to execute a play or perform a skill, he or she is envisioning that play or skill done perfectly. So as athletes develop and improve their skills, they come closer to doing them perfectly. Eventually they will become able to perform more and more of them exactly right.

Moreover, an experienced, skilled athlete will have a finer, more exact understanding of what would be "perfect" for any given play or skill than a beginner. This is natural—as your skills develop, so does your appreciation of what it really takes to get the job done and execute moves and plays to a high standard. Champions actually do execute many moves and skills perfectly—something only they can define for themselves.

This brings us to the idea of *absolute perfection*. This would be the theoretical ability to perform every single movement and skill of every game or performance perfectly—and have all judges, referees, coaches, and teammates agree on it! This is such an incredibly high level of performance or ability in any sport that few athletes come anywhere close to it. But it is definitely something to aim for, and true champions keep themselves moving toward it. Remember that now and then an athlete comes along who performs so spectacularly or breaks so many records that his or her performance is actually said to have been "perfect." Bob Beamon's world-record long jump in the 1968 Olympic Games (which stood for twenty-three years) is one example and, more recently, swimmer Michael Phelps's eight gold medals for eight races in the 2008 Beijing Summer Olympics is another. Also, from decade to decade, performances improve and records are beaten so that the *standard* of perfection in many sports is surpassed and a new one takes its place. And all these broken records are likely results of perfecting all the little things (skills and pieces of those skills) that allow an athlete to compete and/or play the game. The little things *do* matter.

You can see now that "absolute perfection" is not a practical, everyday goal—but a long-term *ideal* (a standard of perfection, a level to be aimed at) that helps keep athletes expanding and increasing their abilities and beating their own past performances. True champions always know that if they strive and give it their all, they can improve their ability beyond its present level, moving up *toward* the ideal of absolute perfection.

On the other hand, true champions don't become too frustrated, too anxious, or feel defeated each time they are unable to achieve "perfection" or a "perfect execution." They are able to accept that they are human, which means that they make mistakes and cannot always do things perfectly. A helpful and practical way to look at practice and training is, rather than constantly trying to do everything perfectly, to always try to execute the skill or play *better* than you did last time, and in this way keep improving it, step by step.

WINNING AND LOSING

My perspective on winning and losing may be quite different from any you have heard before this, so hang on for the ride!

The attitude you have about winning and losing plays a very important role in the development of a mind-set that will lead to increasing excellence. Many athletes, coaches, and even parents today place too much importance on whether a game or competition is won or lost. Winning a particular game or competition becomes the number-one goal (even though it is a short-term objective), and one tends to lose the perspective that, in reality, winning is merely an outcome of good training and practice.

Remember the story about John Wooden? He was a man, a master coach, who viewed winning in this manner. And as you already know, he certainly won his fair share of games and championships—*consecutive* national championships, I might add.

It is a fact that many competitions are either won or lost long before the team or individual ever steps onto the playing field. That is not to say that strategy and decision making during the game are not important, but just that many aspects of strategy and decision making during the game are not under your control, while efforts in training and practice are. Great strategy and decision making during games can never make up for poor performance skills on the part of the players. But training and practice can be done well before the game—*this* is where competitors work on and improve their future performance. So, as I stated earlier, it is on training and practice that you should place your primary focus, since this is where higher levels of performance are actually achieved.

Anyone who places winning as the number-one priority not only loses the correct perspective, as explained above, but also tends to focus too much attention directly on defeating their opponent. This can cause misdirection of an athlete's attention away from the proper goal of training—to develop the athlete's ultimate athletic potential—and onto training that will only allow them to win the next game. This is a situation of diminishing returns because an athlete's *potential*, your potential, may actually be much higher than the level of skill it takes to be successful in any one competition. As a result the athlete, by focusing on this short-term objective (winning), will be undertraining and not working toward his or her ultimate potential.

Additionally, an athlete, by the time of any particular competition, may still not be good enough to defeat the opponent—but that does *not* mean he or she is not on track with their long-term goals and development! Placing so much importance on winning each competition and always making it your primary goal can therefore make it seem you're not doing well enough and deflate your confidence, even when your long-term training is on track and there is no valid reason for feeling bad.

Winning can become such a tight focus for some that they would rather win against a lesser opponent than compete against a stronger one. On several occasions I have heard athletes (and some coaches) discuss their hope that the "star" on another team won't show up for one reason or another, or that a team or individual will lose so they don't have to compete against them—or that their opponent will compete poorly, giving them the better chance at winning.

These attitudes are cop-outs. Any athlete worth the name would much prefer to compete against the *best* athletes when they are *at* their best. The true champion derives little if any satisfaction from any achievement that occurs as a result of an opponent's misfortune or some chance occurrence that gives him or her the advantage. A win like that is tainted.

Successful athletes need to compete against competitors whose skills are at or above their own level. How else can they get a true sense of where they are in relation to what they want to ultimately achieve? Therefore, champions' efforts should center on challenging themselves in this manner—competing against as-good or better opponents.

Now, I am not suggesting that champions should like or accept losing. In fact, they hate it! But they should use it as a motivator for their goal setting, work ethic, and training. A champion knows full well that someone must win and someone must lose. So a champion looks at any loss as a measure of his or her level of achievement or progress at that particular moment (in terms of their skills and everything it takes for them to compete well). And champions look at a win as an outcome of putting forth the right amount of effort in the right places. In each case, they will direct their attention and effort toward what is next on the road to reaching their potential (meaning their next objective or level of skill or achievement).

As we have seen, the importance of winning *and* losing cannot be overstated—*because a champion does not become a champion without experiencing both.*

YOUR SUPPORT SYSTEM

A support system consists of people who help you through technical problems, tough mental and emotional times, and moral and ethical dilemmas. It also may include those who can provide financial support. No matter how knowledgeable, confident, committed, and determined you might be, there is no substitute for the benefits of having a good support system. It is not that an athlete is unable to accomplish what he or she wants without one, but that it is a *lot* easier with this kind of encouragement and assistance.

My support system during my gymnastics career centered on my family. I felt their impact most often through the moral and emotional backing they gave me, when needed, and it was nice to know they always believed I could accomplish my goals. Some athletes are not lucky enough to have these kinds of strong family ties. In fact, there are athletes who have become successful in spite of very difficult and strenuous family structures or even no family structure at all. Usually, however, these people find a coach, friends, or someone else who takes the place of their family and helps them along the way.

In any case, having someone to help support you is an important piece of the puzzle that cannot be overlooked. It is inevitable that competitors will have ups and downs throughout their athletic endeavors. The lows, whether technical or emotional, can really make sports training tough to handle alone. Having someone who really knows you, who understands what you are trying to accomplish, and who really cares about you as a person and has your best interests at heart can really be of benefit through those rough times.

Any individual trying to reach high levels of athletic performance may need to seek out this kind of support if it does not come or occur naturally. Parents and family members are usually the best place to start. However, as mentioned, coaches and friends can also be an important place to go for athletic help and support.

It will be very worthwhile for you to find and build a support system for yourself using what you have available to you. Without one, things can be much more difficult, and it can often be much harder to achieve your goals.

TAKING ACTION

Exercise 1: Reflection on Mind-Set

Your thoughts and answers in this exercise will guide you toward establishing the type of mind-set you need in order to succeed athletically. Take a few moments to reflect on your past experiences (and future possibilities) in the sport you enjoy most. While doing this, think about these three aspects:

1. What would it take for you to feel confident enough that you would "want the ball when the game is on the line"?

2. How much responsibility have you taken upon yourself to improve in that sport you love so much? Have you ever

shunned this responsibility and shifted it onto someone or something else? If so, are you willing to make the changes necessary and take back the responsibility for your improvement and success?

3. What has your own attitude been about winning and losing? Have you placed "winning" as a higher priority than seeking to reach your potential? If yes, how did it make you feel if you lost?

Exercise 2: Your Strengths and Weaknesses

Let's practice applying the principle discussed in the section about strengths and weaknesses.

1. Take out a blank piece of paper and make two columns by drawing a line down the middle of the paper.

2. At the top of the left column write the word *Strengths*, and at the top of the right column write the word *Weaknesses*.

3. Under the left column write down the areas that you consider are the real strengths of your "game" in the sport you participate in. These should be skills or aspects that you are closest to mastering and that you rely on, or lean toward using most often, when you compete.

4. Under the right column write down the skills or aspects that you consider are your weaker areas. These will be the ones you shy away from in competition and that you may not enjoy spending time practicing.

Leave nothing undecided. Place all skills and aspects of your "game" on one side of the line or other. If you have trouble doing this on anything, then base your final decision on whether you like practicing that skill or aspect, and place the "liked" skills on the left under "Strengths" and the "disliked" skills on the right under "Weaknesses."

Take a good look at this list. What you see represents the list of skills that you must master (the left column), and the list of skills you need to transform from weaknesses into strengths (the right column).

By completing this exercise you will have begun laying the foundations for the mind-set you will need to succeed athletically. This, however, is only the beginning.

Chapter 8

Separate yet Related

Mind-Sets for Training and Competition

$\mathcal{A}$t this point you are probably saying to yourself, "Wait, that can't be it! There has to be more to athletic mind-set than this—?" If those are your thoughts, they would be absolutely correct. There *is* more, a lot more.

THE IMPORTANCE OF FOCUS AND CONCENTRATION

The final concept that is part of having a sound mind-set deals with your ability to *focus in on the right areas* at *practice*, and also during *competition*. As a competitive athlete, you will find that there are some distinct differences between these two areas when it comes to correct focus. Developing a good understanding of where your concentration should be during each activity is what this chapter is all about, as knowing this can greatly improve your chances for continued improvement.

I cover *focus* as part of "mind-set" because *focus is the thought process that will guide your actions.* This is very important; it is the difference between guiding your practice so as to give yourself the greatest benefits from it—day by day, long term, and in competition—or practicing randomly with no plan or purpose so that any benefits you gain occur haphazardly or accidentally. Focus makes improvement and progress toward your goals occur as efficiently and predictably as possible.

In Section II, "Building the Dream—The Training Process," you will learn an overall framework or structure for training that you can use to move yourself toward the achievement of your athletic goals. As you carry out your training by following this process, the *specific* things on which you will need to focus and concentrate your efforts will become clear. You'll also discover that in general, while there will be more things to focus on during practice than when competing, some of the things you *need* to concentrate on in competition will be learned during and *through* your training and practice.

Yes, that is correct. There will be fewer things for you to concentrate on when you are competing than when training. This may at first sound strange, but it is true. And yes, these things you concentrate on in competition will be learned through what you focus on in practice. Read on to discover exactly how this all works.

FOCUS AND CONCENTRATION
IN TRAINING AND PRACTICE

Generally, there are three basic purposes or objectives of practice:

1. perfecting current skills and strategies,
2. learning new skills and strategies, and
3. fixing technical problems.

While working on any of these broad areas, you will need to narrow your focus in certain ways. Let me walk you through an example of how this can be applied to practice sessions.

In practice, you will need to focus on breaking down concepts and skills into their most basic and fundamental parts so that each part can be isolated and improved. This is how you will determine your level of achievement—how high you can push your skill.

To accomplish this, you must *visualize* how any component, skill, strategy, or play you are working on should look. You need to see it in your mind's eye. Whether this vision or mental picture comes from videotape, a coach's explanation, or seeing it done correctly by another athlete is not important. What is important is just that you get a good sense or vision of what the skill should look like when it is performed well. Without this vision, your chances of accomplishing the level of skill performance or mastery you are seeking are much less.

When I was training in gymnastics, I knew exactly how I wanted each skill I was working on to look, and it was this mental picture that my efforts were directed toward. This will hold true for any sport where coordinated skills or athletic movements must be learned and performed. Throwing or catching a pass in football, hitting a ball in tennis or golf, and/or shooting baskets in basketball all fall under this same category, and having a solid mental picture of these movements only enhances your ability to acquire and perfect them.

The next step is for you to try to perform the skill being worked on in the same manner as you visualized it, focusing on the feelings and signals the body gives you as the skill is performed. These signals are critical to the learning and perfecting process of any skill (as well as the competitive process, which I will discuss later). If what you are trying to accomplish is done correctly and feels right, you will want to assimilate those signals and feelings into memory so the movement can be repeated. It is just as important for an athlete to *feel* what he or she is doing as it is to *do* it.

This feeling of signals is called "kinesthetic awareness" and/or "proprioceptive awareness." These two terms deal with knowing where the body and its parts are in relation to the space they occupy and in relation to each other while you are performing any particular skill or movement of your sport. These words are a bit tough to use; a simpler term I use for these specific awarenesses is "feel"-type training.

During this whole process of "feel"-type training, you will notice that a few very specific signals really improve your ability to perform well. You should focus your primary attention on these signals as you continue training any skill, for they are the ones that will eventually lead you up the path toward mastery.

To bring some reality to these concepts, here is a specific example of how this all works. Take volleyball spiking. One of the first things a player must learn is how to correctly approach the ball for a spike before he or she can leave the ground and properly execute this skill. Learning this will take many repetitions before the body picks up the coordination behind it and the movement becomes natural. Using the "feel"-type training concepts just discussed, the athlete would concentrate on the actual leg, feet, arm, and body movements while practicing the approach and would pick up on the physical signals the body is giving him or her. The athlete should only focus on the specific cues that *enhance* the performance of this skill, and repeat them, while all others are discarded. As the player improves, he or she will learn and be able to replicate the correct form much faster *with* this focus than just going through the motions of doing approaches *without* this focus.

This same idea can be used to learn new skills (like the one just mentioned), to execute new movements in sports like basketball or football, or to improve or perfect skills you already have. You can (1) literally break down the skill into parts (working on them one at a time), or (2) you can direct your attention to one area of that skill each time you perform it. Whichever way you use the concept of focus, the result will be the same: you will experience a faster, more efficient, and better-quality improvement of athletic performance.

This concept of focus in training is one of those little things that can make a *big* difference, and it is what many athletes do NOT take the time or effort to do. It is a much easier path to just go through the motions mindlessly or automatically than to concentrate your attention and efforts in this manner, but it is effort well spent.

And remember, almost all of the principles I discussed earlier—determination, commitment, discipline, sacrifice, heart, knowing your strengths and weaknesses, striving toward perfection—will also play a key role in your ability to narrow and concentrate your focus during *training*.

I also want to remind you of what I said in chapter 3 about desire:

You really have to want to accomplish something in order to have any chance at achieving

it. Desire breeds passion, and passion supports, develops, and strengthens *commitment*, *discipline*, *sacrifice*, and the setting of your priorities.

Part of this desire comes from *enjoying* your ability to perform skills, movements, and techniques, or to run plays in such a manner that it feels smooth, solid, and effortless. Using kinesthetic and proprioceptive signals for training, as explained just above, is what creates this opportunity. As I have said, it is difficult to put into words the fulfillment, self-satisfaction, and fun you can have when you can perform in this way. Taking pride in this ability builds a passion to repeat it, and this becomes another cyclical pattern of success feeding upon success that leads you upward toward true championship.

THE DIFFERENCE BETWEEN FOCUS IN TRAINING AND FOCUS IN COMPETITION

During competitions, an athlete will need to shift his or her focus from one of *correction, learning, and perfecting* (as discussed in detail above) to one of *execution of performance*. Competitors must direct their attention this way in order to have the greatest chance of doing their best when they compete. Anything dealing with *development* or *major correction* needs to be left in the gym or on the practice field. Once you hit the competitive arena, it is time to relax and let the body perform what it has learned.

One of the purposes and advantages of training using kinesthetic and proprioceptive signals ("feel"-type training) is that, once learned, they can be used naturally, without conscious thought, during competition. This type of focus allows you to keep things simple—and keeping things simple enables concentration only on what will give you the best performance. For example, if a pitcher in baseball is working on a curve, at some point during the training of this pitch he will start to get the movement he wants out of the ball (just like the volleyball player got the coordination of the approach in the example given earlier). As the pitcher moves along the learning curve, he will want to feel exactly what his body is doing. He will want to feel

- the movement of his legs and arms as he starts his motion and strides forward,

- how his body feels as his hips and shoulders turn and accelerate into the pitch,

- where his elbow is in relation to his shoulder,

- how relaxed his arm is as he starts it moving,

- the lightness of his grip on the ball along with how his fingers lie across the seams, and

- the sensation he gets as the ball snaps off his hand and heads toward home plate.

Eventually the pitcher will get to the point where he is able to execute this pitch so consistently that he can add it to his repertoire of pitches. During the game, when the catcher calls for this pitch, the pitcher should draw upon the kinesthetic and proprioceptive signals he learned in practice—especially the few specific signals that truly make this pitch work for him. He should *relax* and use these signals to emulate the same motion he achieved in training. As his curve continues to improve, so will the strength of these signals—and he will be able to *know exactly* what his body is doing. In due time, the pitch will become repeatable without the pitcher even having to think about it. The pitcher will know long before his curve ever crosses the plate whether it was good or not, just by how it feels. The pitch has been so well trained that he feels as if he could throw it in his sleep.

It is possible that you may have experienced something like this with skills you are already doing very well. Think about it for a

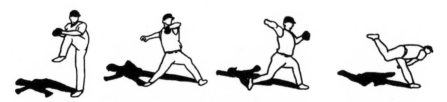

8.1: "FEEL" the Pitch

moment. Have you ever performed a skill in a game or competition and known, without a doubt, that it was going to be "good" just by how your body movements felt as you executed that skill? If so, you have some idea of what we have been discussing. If not, putting forth strong effort to work on your skill set (all of your skills) in the manner in which I have described, along with following the guidelines I detail in Section II, will certainly make that possible.

This whole process of learning during training and using it in competition is actually a progression. The difference is only in the shift of focus from *learning* these signals (during training) to *repeating signals already learned* (during competition). This shift in concentration will make a *big* difference on how successful you are at performing skills and techniques in competitive situations. Realize that using your senses *in practice* when developing a new skill or when perfecting a skill is not the same way you use your senses in competition. In training you are focused on *learning* these signals and trying to figure out the correct execution. But bringing that type of mind-set into competition can detract from your ability to do your best and can be an underlying factor in why some athletes choke when the pressure is on.

The reason is simple to understand. It is very difficult, if not impossible, to perform well if the athlete is concerning himself with correcting technical problems or trying to refine skills (or strategies) in a competitive situation. Doing that causes a misdirection of focus. In competition you don't get a second chance to repeat anything in order to make it better. Instead, athletes really need to focus their attention on kinesthetic and proprioceptive senses *already developed and ingrained in their memory*. This allows skills, strategies, and/or plays to be performed at peak levels.

Another advantage to focusing on these learned sensory signals in competition is that the ability to do so allows athletes to block out unwanted stimuli that can easily distract them from their objective. Being able to block out unwanted stimuli by focusing on your own learned sensory signals increases your chances of higher levels of performance.

Now, there will be instances, especially with strategies or plays in team sports, where you cannot entirely rely on already-learned skills and movements. Say, for example, a team is not performing well because of the strategy they are using in a game. They may have to make adjustments to this strategy and change to a different strategy that they have not practiced well. Even with a change like this, however, the athlete will still have to rely on his or her basic skills to be able to perform well, so using the principle explained above will increase his or her chances for success.

VISUALIZATION DURING COMPETITION

Visualization is a tool that not only pays big dividends for the training athlete, as discussed earlier, but for the competing athlete as well. Do you think it is possible for you—or any athlete—to be successful if you cannot see yourself succeeding? I am not sure you can—at least not consistently. It is a common practice of successful athletes to visualize their performance at its best before they actually compete.

During competition, you should always try to envision how you want to perform. My own practice before competition was to run through the most important parts of my (gymnastics) ring routine in my mind, making sure everything was visualized to its completion exactly as I thought it should be done. I would even move my arms in the same manner as I would move them when I was competing.

This same type of visualization can be used in any sport. Whether you are executing a play in football or soccer or performing a figure skating routine—or even preparing yourself for a wrestling match—seeing in your mind how you want everything to go is a big, positive step toward making it happen.

PRESSURE AND INTENSITY IN COMPETITION

The competitive arena is not a very forgiving place. Just its nature brings a level of intensity not found during the athlete's training process. Not only do successful competitors learn to deal effectively with this intensity, they actually thrive in it. The more pressure they feel, the better they seem to perform. The reason behind this centers

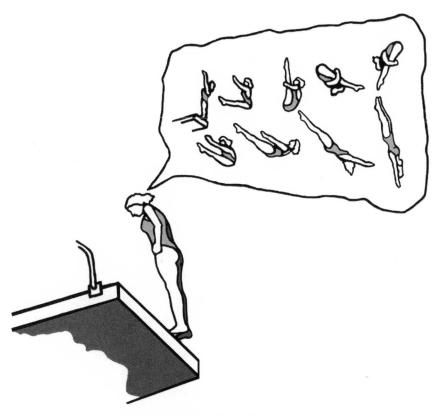

8.2: In Your "Mind's Eye"

on learning to control this intensity rather than letting the intensity, and the adrenaline that comes with it, take control of you.

This controlled intensity you are looking for is achieved through concentration (focus) on whatever the task is at hand. Being misdirected by allowing yourself to get so worked up during competition that you cannot function efficiently or effectively is of no help to your mind-set. Any competitor will be able to move quicker, faster, throw farther and harder, and jump higher than they might in practice because of the adrenaline rush that occurs in competition. This increased ability can actually hinder their performance if a conscious effort is not made to control it. Bringing 100 percent *relaxed* attention to those few inner and ingrained signals that you learned during training (the kinesthetic and proprioceptive, "feel"-type signals we discussed earlier) will be of great benefit here. Then you just take a deep breath, relax, and let your body do its thing. This is regardless of the score, intensity of the competition, time left on the clock, environment you are in, or how large the crowd is. These are all irrelevant to what you must do to perform at your best.

Take two softball pitchers, both capable of sixty-mph fastballs. One of these pitchers tends to focus on trying to throw that ball as hard as she can while the other concentrates on relaxing, letting her body flow, and seeing where that strike zone is. Now, pit them against each other in the finals of an NCAA championship game—who would you put your money on? Which one will use the increased pressure and intensity to her advantage, and which one will allow this intensity to govern her pitching and thus have a tendency toward becoming wild and unpredictable? If you said that the second pitcher—the one who concentrates on relaxing, letting her body flow, and finding that strike zone—will have the advantage, you are right.

I can remember one specific example from my high school gymnastics experience, where I tried to execute my first two skills as rapidly and powerfully as I could, thinking this would improve my score. Needless to say, my routine was all over the place. The power and speed were definitely there, but the control was gone. I learned very quickly that without control over this intensity (and adrenaline), athletic performance becomes very uncertain. The more intense the competition, the more focused you will need to be in order to use the intensity to your advantage.

My normal procedure, after experiencing that situation above, was to take a couple of deep, smooth, relaxed breaths (and I actually said "relax" to myself mentally). I would then bring my focus to bear on visualizing my skills done "perfectly" using the kinesthetic and proprioceptive signals I had trained with. If I felt myself becoming tense, I just repeated this procedure using my key word, *relax*, as I continued visualizing my performance. This worked well for me all through my competitive years no matter what the level of competition I was in. You, too, could benefit from such a strategy. All you need to do is discover for yourself what key word or words work best for you and then use the procedure that I explained above.

Another way of learning to deal with this type of competitive pressure is to try to bring as much of it into your *training sessions* as possible. This can be accomplished through mock competitive situations you create for yourself during practice. It is a mental game you play, using your imagination. It usually takes the form of creating or imagining "do or die" type situations, such as making the last shot in basketball with one second left, or a 3-and-2 pitch count with the game on the line, or performing your last dive, which needs to be perfect in order to win.

This may also be accomplished by setting a specific number of skill repetitions (or completions of performance) and not moving on in your training until they are all performed at a high level of execution—and you can get similar results every time.

A third strategy would be to set up practice so that you are always competing against someone, or *for* something. If you have a coach, however, he or she will normally set this up by creating various drills and adverse competitive situations where the winners of these competitive situations are rewarded in some manner. The whole idea here is to put more pressure on yourself during training with the hope that it will bring big benefits to you during competition. The closer to competition you can make practice feel, the easier it will be for you to handle the pressure that arises in the athletic arena.

YOUR ATTITUDE TOWARD YOUR COMPETITORS

Up to this point, my explanation of focus as it relates to the competitive mind-set has centered on you, the athlete. Little, if anything, has been mentioned about the competitors. The reason for this goes back to something I have alluded to more than a few times—*the things the athlete has control over* and *those he or she does not have control over*. It does not matter how good athletes become, they will never have control over how fast, how strong, or how good their opponents are. *Therefore, focusing on the opponents does nothing but distract you from your purpose.*

Teams and individuals who do not understand this end up playing down to the level of their competitors, or losing to competitors they could beat, instead of performing consistently closer to their own potential. On numerous occasions I have witnessed a team's inability to perform any higher or better than the competition they are against. It is probable you have seen this happen as well, or maybe even experienced it as a member of a team that was playing poorly against an opponent you knew your team was better than.

Well, the longer an athlete or team continues to focus on their competitors and what *they* are doing (over which they have no control), the more likely they will continue to play at that same poor level. You must aim *higher* than your opponents, and you do that by staying focused on what *you* need to execute in competition, in addition to training to reach your own highest potential. This concept holds true for most competitive activities, with the exception of just a few sports.

Athletic activities in which you compete directly against an opponent give the illusion that you must focus on what they are doing (or might do) and that *their behavior* should dictate what you do next. This is an extremely common misconception. Sports like wrestling and tennis, as well as the majority of team sports, fit into this category. But this is actually a half-truth at best, or, better stated, a misplaced perception of concentration. In such sports, it is just as important for athletes to try to put as much control as possible over what happens on the competitive floor into their own hands.

Exerting control over your opponent can be accomplished by *using an offensive strategy* and, by doing so, *dictating for your competitors* what *they* will do! Serving to the weaker stroke of an opponent in tennis, pulling on a wrestler's arm during a match in order to get him to shift his weight to where you want it, and running a play to the weaker side of a team you are competing against (in just about any team sport) are all examples of how you can control your opponent by taking the offense.

Then, in response to anything that an adversary does offensively or strategically (any tactic an opponent uses against you), or when anything unpredictable happens, you should just react and adapt to it as a natural part of the game by relying on the sound fundamentals and strategies you (and your team) have developed during practice.

So you see that what you, the competitor, set your focus on is all in the perspective you take. The opponent is really just another part of the environment that you face while competing. Since you cannot change the environment, you must either adapt to it or take control over it by what you, the athlete, decide to do. Again, the best perspective is to focus on what *you* need to do, *not* on what your opponent might do.

As you continue to train, compete, and improve, you will invariably find yourself in situations during competition that can make it difficult to concentrate. This difficulty may come from another competitor trying to intimidate you. (There are all kinds of mind games that an opponent can play in order to take athletes' minds off their mission. It might be something they say, the intensity they bring into a warm-up or game, or simply their behavior and ability.) Or maybe this inability to concentrate is due to muscle soreness or fatigue from previous training sessions, or you are just getting back from an injury or illness, or you haven't been getting the right amount of sleep lately—or there may even have been some type of emotional trauma. Whatever the reason, the strategies we have covered in this chapter will help you stay focused and on track. Champions are particularly good at overcoming these types of obstacles. They enjoy the confidence they gain through their focused training sessions and use the competitive arena as a measure of their performance along the path toward their goals.

TAKING ACTION

An Exercise in Focus

This exercise will help you better understand how an athlete should try to focus when training and/or competing by demonstrating it to you. It is intended as an example through action and is not necessarily a training tool for improving one's focus.

Find yourself a small ball that bounces fairly well. A golf ball would be perfect for this. You will also need a partner to help you (and a third person would be helpful if someone is available). Now go somewhere that has a hard floor surface the ball can easily bounce off, in a location that holds no safety concerns for anyone involved and contains no objects that could break.

1. Toss the ball maybe one foot or so above your head, straight up, and in front of you, then let it bounce and catch it with two hands. Do this several times with the goal being to just catch the ball each and every time. Easy, right? Not much concentration needed here.

2. Now do the same thing, only this time count "one" out loud the first time you make a catch, "two" the second time, "three" the third time, and so on. Do this ten times with the goal being to catch the ball each and every time, and count up an additional number with every catch.

   A little bit harder, but still easy for you, I'm sure. You may have had to bring a little more concentration and focus into what you were doing, but still not that much more.

3. Now here is where it gets interesting. Have your partner count random numbers out loud while you are trying to accomplish the same thing you just did. Throw the ball up, let it bounce, catch it in two hands, and count up one number for each catch to ten catches as your partner randomly says numbers out loud. Did you find it more difficult to focus?

4. Now try it again, making every effort to relax, and concentrate *only* on the ball and the number you are going to call on each catch. Try to block everything else out, narrowing your focus to just relaxing, catching the ball, and your counting—that is it.

   How did you do? Did you notice the voice of your partner seeming softer than it did the first time and your task becoming more of a focal point for you (meaning the thing you were most aware of)? It may take a little practice before you can identify this, but you should notice this in time.

5. To test this further, use a third person to call out different random numbers at the same time your initial partner does. You can also make the skill more difficult in several other ways: by catching the ball with one hand, by having one of your partners bounce the ball to you as they call out random numbers, or maybe even by catching the ball with one hand, *palm down*, as it bounces up to you off the ground.

However, in all cases, as the task becomes more difficult and/or the distractions increase, you should notice that your level of focus, concentration, and ability to relax will have to increase for you to complete the task as efficiently and easily as you did the first time, when you were just catching the ball with two hands. What you have just experienced is an example of proper focus for the task at hand.

Expectation from Practice

— Improving the *quality* of your practice is all about thinking *outside the box* through increasing what you *expect from yourself.* Expect to learn and improve on today what you could not learn or perform yesterday. Expect to perfect what you practice and expect the absolute best from yourself when you train—nothing less.

Set a certain number of skill repetitions that must be accomplished at the next higher level. Be happy when you accomplish that number and angry when you don't. Remember that giving up on this is not an option, even though you may have to wait until the next day, week, or month to get there. Once there, keep increasing that expectation, that next level of excellence, and that number you want to accomplish: it will be a never-ending struggle that you know ahead of time you must submit yourself to.

Doing this will be the hardest, most frustrating, challenging, and stressful thing that you, the athlete, will have to endure because it will sometimes seem that you work so very hard to get nowhere. But . . .

— It is in doing this that you will be able to reach inside and pull from within the true champion who exists there. It is what will allow you to perform at levels others only dream of and leave people who see you play in awe at your performance—and not once or twice, but *all the time.*

When you train yourself to practice with this type of expectation *every single day*, you will then be able to step onto the competitive field against the very best and most feared athlete in the world, knowing that what he or she brings to the competitive arena will be more difficult than anything you will ever face, yet KNOWING WITHOUT A DOUBT that, in your *worst* moment, your performance will stifle, overshadow, and nullify anything they do.

— It is at that exact moment that you will realize how good you have become and that all the effort you have put in has been worth it.

— "What then?" you may ask.

— Do it all over again!

SECTION II

Building the Dream—
The Training Process

$\mathcal{A}$t this stage, you should have a deeper understanding of how important your thought processes are to seeing your athletic dream come to fruition. So where do we go from here? The answer to that question is up next, as you and I start putting the actual training "pieces" together in preparation for what you will actually be doing at practice.

Everything I have been teaching you, combined with everything you will learn in the coming chapters, will place you in a position where *you* govern what will happen for you. I am about to lay out a workable, easy-to-use *training framework*—an overall long-term plan, structure, or strategy—that you can use to help yourself flourish and succeed in your chosen sport.

Up to this point I have spent a great deal of time talking about the principles that make up a true champion. The reason for this is that these qualities form the foundation for everything else that you will do in the "process" or "work" part of your program—your training.

This whole concept of development from an athlete into a champion is similar in nature to the building of a house. The first thing to do before the construction begins is to develop a plan or vision. For sports, that vision is represented by the GOALS the athlete sets.

The next phase deals with the excavation and pouring of the house's foundation. From my point of view, all other principles discussed in Section I—TAKING RESPONSIBILITY, DESIRE, CDSPH, CHARACTER AND INTEGRITY, ATHLETIC MIND-SET, etc.—make up the rest of this foundation. Just as the rest of the house will only be as strong as the foundation that it sits on, so will your success depend on the foundation you have built of the principles and qualities of a true champion. Add a little bit of pressure or stress to your "house" and, without a strong foundation, everything crumbles. Success becomes just random luck. However, in athletics, just as in construction, once a strong foundation has been laid, assembly can start on the building phase. This is represented in athletics through the training framework you will put together and follow during practice.

Chapter 9

From the Ground Up

Fundamentals for Success

Fundamentals are the most basic and primary elements and skills of any sport or athletic activity, as well as the basic movements of any specific skill or trick an athlete performs.

$\mathscr{I}$ know you have heard the term *fundamentals* before; we briefly discussed it in chapter 1, only I left out all the details. In this chapter we will fill in those details, moving you closer toward accomplishing your athletic goals.

As discussed in the introduction to this section, a *training framework* is a training strategy or training outline—a plan of what you are going to do at practice. You decide on this framework, or overall long-term plan, based on the techniques and skills you will need to learn and master to achieve your goals. It is during this training process that you will spend the most time, energy, and physical effort.

Forming the backbone of this framework is the development of strong fundamentals. It is the *fundamentals* that form the basis or foundation for all further learning. Mastering fundamentals is the cornerstone of any progression or improvement.

I am sure you have seen very young children learning to walk, right? You notice how unsteady they are when trying to take their first few steps, wobbling here and there, falling forward onto their hands or backward onto their behinds. At this stage, they haven't quite developed the *fundamental* balance and coordination to just get up and walk like you and I do. However, as these two fundamentals become stronger through the many efforts they exert in trying to walk, eventually they do learn to walk.

Now, how silly would it be to take a young child who has not yet gained the fundamental balance and coordination needed to walk, stand them at the top of a hill, and expect them to run down that hill as their momentum started to carry them forward. That's a disaster waiting to happen. However, there are many athletes who are essentially doing the same thing by trying to accomplish more difficult skills or techniques than they have yet built the foundations for.

Fundamentals are, unfortunately, something that many tend to forget as they move along their path of athletic experience. An athlete may put together the best competitive strategy possible, yet it will be worthless without the fundamentals to carry it out. As a parent and former coach, I have seen so many athletes end up sacrificing their basic skills, their *fundamentals*, in their sport in order to develop strategies for playing the game. It is amazing to see how much time athletes and teams spend practicing some play or attempting some skill that they have little chance of accomplishing well, consistently, or under pressure, because they lack the fundamentals to achieve it.

The approach you should be taking to acquire your fundamentals (all skills, actually) centers on the use of *progressions*—a gradual method for learning and physical achievement in which one ability or skill is built upon the previous (somewhat like climbing a set of stairs, step by step), until you eventually reach a point of peak performance. You, the athlete, must learn to walk before you can run, yet too many spend too much time on strategies and skills they are not ready to attempt. There are coaches and parents who are inadvertently guilty of promoting and supporting this idea (usually because of their overemphasis on "trying" to win), so you should remain aware of this possible stumbling block.

Let's use soccer as an example to further explain the use of progressions to learn fundamentals. The game uses plays and strategies such as overlaps, making runs, crossing, etc. An enormous amount of time can be spent practicing these plays and strategies. In fact, most if not all of a practice can be taken up by scrimmage-type work like this. Yet if the players on a team that spends most of its time practicing the above types of tactics cannot first trap, pass, and kick a ball accurately and efficiently (three mandatory basics of soccer), it is unlikely they will be able to execute these strategies well or consistently—or *any* strategy, for that matter.

I am not suggesting that no time during practice should be spent on learning the strategies of the game. But I am suggesting that you should spend much more time and effort on learning and perfecting your fundamentals. If this is not a feasible option based on the practice time available, then it is one of those things that you must find time to do on your own. In fact, no matter what level an athlete has reached, working on these skills should always be an integral part of his or her training. (In my own career, I believed this to be so important that much of my training focused on perfecting fundamentals. You'll see why, and how it benefited me, as you read through "Putting It All Together—A True Story" in Section III.)

Take two teams, equally matched, and put them in competition against each other in a championship game and invariably the team that will come out on top consistently will be the one with the strongest fundamentals. I have even seen lesser athletes or teams succeed over more-talented ones because they were stronger in their "basics" than their opponents. This is why I cannot emphasize mastering one's fundamentals strongly enough. The *fundamental skills or basics are the foundation for everything else that will be performed.* So, this is another one of those "little things" that can make the difference between success and failure.

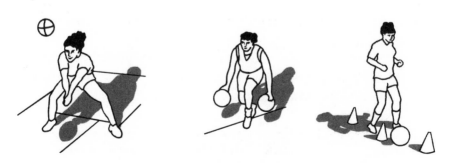

9.1: The "Fundamental" Difference

TWO TYPES OF FUNDAMENTALS

I like to divide fundamentals into two general categories, with both of them taking precedence over the strategies used to "win" games. The first category consists of *the basic components and skills needed to perform efficiently* in the athlete's sport. The second fundamental in any sport deals with *the basic strategic movements used within that sport.*

1. Basic Skills of the Sport

Take the still rings event in gymnastics, for example. A gymnast will need to be able to swing efficiently, hold a solid handstand, develop good air sense for dismounting, and be physically strong in a variety of positions. As the gymnast develops ability in these areas and starts to really improve, some of these fundamentals will change and may even be combined to form one skill. The basic swing and the handstand will be combined into a swing to handstand. For ringmen at higher levels, this combination would be a basic. A gymnast might actually increase his fundamental list by working on a swing to handstand, in practice, and then a handstand by itself, as a separate entity, during the conditioning portion of his training. This is only one very specific example of some fundamentals and how some of them might be trained.

Again, let's use soccer to apply this same "basic skills" concept in a team sport. Some fundamentals here include basic forms of trapping, passing, ball handling, and shooting. These four skills are an integral part of being able to play this game. Without them, an athlete is merely playing kickball. Just as in the gymnastic example, these skills may change slightly or be combined, but they should never be forgotten and should always be a major part of a soccer player's training. In fact, these skills should be trained to the extent that a player can confidently accomplish them without any conscious thought—*something that holds true for any sport or activity in which you want to reach excellence.*

Additionally, any skill (whether basic or advanced) that you, the athlete, perform will have fundamental components to it that you must execute in order to accomplish that skill. For example, a volleyball player needs to learn how to approach, jump, and swing his or her arm correctly before being able to perform a spike. Tennis players need to learn the proper stance, grip, ball toss, and arm swing before being able to serve properly. Basketball players need to be balanced, have their eyes on the basket, their shooting elbow under the ball, and have good follow-through on their shot in order to shoot correctly. All of these components are considered basic and fundamental to these skills.

Now, I do not pretend to know every basic skill or fundamental for every sport, and even if my knowledge base did include them, it would be impossible to list them all here. The basic idea for me to get across to you here is how essential these fundamentals are.

Discover and build your own list of fundamental skills for your own sport. Then develop a training plan that includes them.

2. Basic Strategies Used in the Sport

The second type of fundamental in any sport deals with the basic strategies used in that activity. Now, do not confuse this with the development of a game plan intended to defeat the opponent—this is not the same thing. Here I am talking about the basic and fundamental movements of the athlete on the field of play, or the strategies used when putting together a performance, such as the sequence of skills that will go into making up the best and most effective gymnastics performance. In tennis this may include the place where a player positions himself or herself when returning the serve, during play, or when volleying at the net. In figure skating it might involve the best way to put together one's performance, deciding which skills go at which time in the routine and which sequence will be more impressive. In soccer or basketball a basic strategy would cover movements that create space in order to set up passing lanes.

All sports contain key strategic concepts and fundamental principles of movement. To learn these, the athlete must become a "student of the game": You must learn by watching others who are successful in your sport, by reading or viewing materials written or supported by experts of the sport, and by talking and listening to people who have the expertise to help you.

Keep in mind that these strategic skills do not take precedence over the "basic skills of the sport"—the fundamental skills explained in the previous section. However, these strategic fundamentals are still essential basic pieces of the "game" and do need to be a center of focus in your training and practice.

I hope that you now understand the great importance of including fundamentals within the framework or core of what you, as an athlete, need to master to attain success. Their worth will be seen most often when everything is on the line and the competitive situations are the toughest. This is when athletes will rely on the strength of their fundamentals to carry them through.

It is essential that you, the competitor, take the initiative to train yourself on whatever the basic skills are within your sport—whether the coach includes them in practice or not. You will need to spend whatever time is necessary to improve and perfect these skills so that you will be able to reach the level of performance you are seeking.

TAKING ACTION

Your Own Fundamentals

While the information from this chapter is still fresh in your mind (and since all sports contain fundamentals), it would be a good idea for you to make a list of *basic* essential skills for the sport you choose to participate in.

1. Take a few moments and write down as many as you can think of, positioning them in the center of the page, leaving room on both the left and right sides of your list (you'll need to use this space in a later exercise). You don't need to develop a comprehensive or complete list here, just one to get you started thinking and moving in the right direction.

2. Now look closely at your list. As you examine it, look for (1) the skills that are the most basic and essential (including the ones needed to even "play the game" at all); (2) those fundamental skills that are the *foundation* for learning and performing more

difficult technical elements—ones that rise above a basic level; and (3) skills that can be broken down into their fundamental parts for training purposes. This is all good mental practice regarding what was taught in this chapter and what will be emphasized in future chapters.

You should find it interesting that much of what you wrote down will fit into all three of these categories!

3. Now keep only three to five of these on your list (the ones you feel are most important), crossing off the rest. Keep this list handy—you will use it in combination with other information a little later in this book.

Remember, we are trying to get you thinking and moving in the right direction and not necessarily having you put together your final training list. Anything you cross off you can add back anytime you choose.

• Chapter 10 •

Pieces and Parts

Breaking It Down

*R*emember the "pieces" I mentioned in the introduction to Section II? Well, in this chapter we will be using that term a little more literally. Many times throughout this book I've talked about how important training is to the attainment of an athlete's goals. The fundamentals discussed in chapter 9 are only one very important aspect of that training.

The next aspect encompasses breaking down an athlete's particular sport or activity into its principal parts. The purpose of this breakdown will be to objectively divide up the sport, event, or activity into areas of concentration or similarity to help you organize your training. It is in this breakdown phase that we really deal with the nuts and bolts of what you, the competitor, will be working on.

It is easiest for me to demonstrate this concept using examples from my own high school athletic experiences.

The first thing I did, and what you will have to do, was to mentally step back from the intricacies of my chosen event, the still rings, in order to get a more objective view. I asked myself this question: "What areas of this event are critical for a gymnast to master to be successful?"

The answer included not only the basic fundamentals of the event, as described in the previous chapter, but also much more difficult and technical skills, strategic ways to put these skills together, and the conditioning or strength needed to perform them.

I then divided these areas into three specific categories:

- swinging movements,
- strength movements, and
- dismounts.

I selected these three broad categories because whenever I observed other great gymnasts performing this event, all were exceptional in these three areas. Doing this helped to simplify a whole range of skills into a more organized and functional format, making it easier to focus my concentration.

I then further divided each group into its principal parts:

1. Swinging movements included
   - various ways to swing to a handstand,
   - the handstand itself,
   - giants (forward and back),
   - dislocates, etc.

2. Strength moves included
   - different presses to a handstand,
   - crosses,
   - malteses, etc.

3. Dismounts included some type of double-back.

This procedure made a fairly complicated training process much more practical and manageable.

Once I had this division of movements, I divided up my practice in the same manner, allocating whatever time was necessary for each one. Some areas were more difficult than others, so more time was spent there. I also carried out extensive conditioning at the end of every training session.

Any sport can be broken down into categories, just like I have above for the still rings event in gymnastics. Take basketball, for example. There are basically three parts to the game:

1. The technical or skill phase, which includes
   - passing,
   - ball handling,
   - dribbling,
   - shooting, etc.

Each of these categories of skills can be broken down further into specific types of skills that are then trained individually *and* as a team. Using passing to illustrate this further breakdown, examples would include a bounce pass, chest pass, overhand pass, one-arm pass, etc.

2. The strategic phase, which includes
   - movement without the ball,
   - individual and team movements or plays (both offensive and defensive),
   - offensive and defensive transitioning, etc.

If a player can also become a student of the game—a concept mentioned in chapter 9, "From the Ground Up"—this will help tremendously in this second area of basketball training.

3. Conditioning to develop the athleticism needed to play the game, which includes
   - strength,
   - sprinting endurance,
   - vertical jump,
   - quickness,
   - agility,
   - speed, etc.

Some of the above will be trained during the skill and strategic phases of a practice, while the rest are emphasized during conditioning.

Even volleyball can be divided into groups in the same manner:

1. The technical or skill phase:
   - overhand and underhand passing,
   - attacking,

- blocking,
- serving,
- practicing serve receive, etc.

2. The strategic phase:
   - court movement, both individual and as a team,
   - offensive and defensive formations, transitioning, and strategies.

3. The conditioning and athletic phase:
   - speed,
   - strength,
   - agility,
   - quickness,
   - vertical jump,
   - anaerobic conditioning, etc.

Again, these examples don't necessarily include every skill or breakdown needed to be successful in basketball or volleyball. However, they should serve to show you in a simple manner how any sport can be broken down to simplify your training. Every athletic activity brings with it a unique set of circumstances, yet all can be categorized in the manner I have described, making practice much more efficient and effective.

ALLOCATING TIME FOR PRACTICE

It would seem, as an athlete continues to improve, that he or she would find it impossible to fit all that needs to be done into one practice session of reasonable length. It looks as though the list of skills—which should also always include some work on fundamentals—would grow to mountainous proportions.

However, this is *not* the case for two reasons. First, in many sports, as an athlete reaches higher levels of performance and competition, he or she tends to specialize in certain areas of the game, sport, or event, so the skills they need become specific to the position they are concentrating on or the level they have reached. For example, outside hitters in volleyball will concentrate more on passing and hitting, while setters will spend most of their time on overhand passing (setting). It is not that they stop training in other aspects of the game, but just that more emphasis and time will be spent in their particular area of focus—so they don't have to devote an equal amount of time to the areas outside their specialty. In addition, as athletes become more accomplished, they become more selective in the skills they know they need to spend the most time on—the ones that truly make the most difference in increasing their chances for success.

The second reason there should be time for everything you need to work on is that most successful athletes use a form of combination training, where skills are combined or grouped, including fundamentals (as mentioned briefly in chapter 9). Examples would include a gymnast combining several skills together, rather than working on each one, one at a time; an outside hitter in volleyball who passes a served ball to the setter, then immediately moves into a hitting position, spiking the ball after the setter sets her pass; or a basketball player performing a three-point shot, a jump shot a little closer to the basket, and a layup, all in succession. This not only decreases the actual time the athlete spends, making training more efficient, it also makes practice a little more like competition, thus increasing its effectiveness.

Furthermore, on skills that you have truly started to master, you can add the dimension of practicing these skills against an opponent to further create competitive scenarios that mirror what you will see in the competitive arena.

The more your practice resembles the "game," the easier it will be to perform in that game. Working smarter, not harder, is an important concept that competitive athletes need to apply if they ever want to get out of the gym or off the practice field. All that said, however, a true champion will likely always find something he or she wants to spend more time on so that its consistency and effectiveness can be maintained or improved.

TECHNICAL INFORMATION

I would be remiss if I did not take a little more time to talk about where you can obtain the technical information you need to enable you to learn and perfect the skills and fundamentals involved in your particular activity. For many, a lot of this information will come from your coach, as will some of the training we have been discussing. However, there are other excellent sources you can use to supplement your knowledge and enhance your learning potential.

One great way a motivated athlete can acquire this information is through attending summer camps and clinics or joining clubs. All of these can be great places to pick up strategies for improving your skills and learning new things.

The coaches at many clubs and summer camps, along with the college athletes attending or helping out at these camps, are some of the best in their field. Their teachings will provide you with immeasurable assistance. The same can be said for clinics, which are shorter in duration and cover more specific areas than camps. Many club- or college-level coaches run these.

In addition to the teaching received as part of the camp or clinic programs, making personal contact with these individuals for advice can be a big help to competitors if they plan to compete at the collegiate level. You should not hesitate to do so for fear they will not want to be bothered with you; these professionals are as interested in meeting serious up-and-coming athletes as you are in meeting them.

Last, books, videotapes, DVDs, and the Internet are all good sources of technical information. You can also get information directly from teammates and other athletes by critically watching them train and perform, and even by listening as others are being coached. Personally, I am a visual learner, and much of my information in high school came from watching others train and perform, as well as from listening to coaches teach skills and techniques to other athletes. There is a wealth of good information out there, as long as you are willing to take the time and make the effort to seek it out.

During this process of finding technical information, you should keep in mind several important points. First, make sure to look for experts in your particular activity or sport. No matter whose training and learning vehicle(s) you choose, all should have proven track records of success or, in the case of books and videotapes, their authors should be successful coaches and/or athletes. When you find a potential source of technical information, find out what other athletes have achieved with it. Successful coaches, camps, and clubs tend to "breed" other successful athletes, and they usually do it consistently over time. This is also true for books and/or DVDs and videotapes by successful coaches and athletes—their information and methods should have helped others improve, so see if you can find athletes who can vouch for the book or video.

Second, even with all the emphasis above on finding sources that have been proven reliable and successful, don't be afraid to think outside the box and develop logical strategies and techniques for gaining technical knowledge for yourself that may go against the so-called norms of your sport. Sometimes traveling an unconventional path can bring rewards and accomplishments not thought possible. Any method you can use to find valuable knowledge about your sport, if it is technically sound and it works for you, is valid.

Last, be patient with your efforts when using new or different techniques for improving your skills or performance. Often you will go backward and seem to get worse before you see any improvement (this is not always the case, but it is fairly usual). When you force the body—or mind, for that matter—to do something that it's not used to doing, it tends to follow the path of least resistance. This usually encompasses previously learned motor patterns and movements. It can be very difficult to break these patterns so, again, be patient with yourself. If the technique is correct and you can persevere through this difficult phase, improvements will come.

TAKING ACTION

Your Own Skills and Technical Elements

Just as we did at the end of chapter 9, where you created a list of basic skills (fundamentals), I would like you to make an additional list from your sport of choice. However, this time choose three to five skills or technical elements that are *above* the basic level and that you can already perform (but may need improvement on) or skills/ technical elements that you still want or need to learn. Write them down the center of the page as you did the fundamentals.

Most of these skills should build on the foundations developed from practice on your fundamentals and may even be advanced versions of these basic skills. As with the list from chapter 9, keep this list available for your use in the exercises following chapter 11.

A brief example for a beginning/intermediate volleyball player might include the following (I have first created a fundamentals list using the concepts taught in chapter 9 so you can see the close connection between the two lists):

Fundamentals list from chapter 9
Forearm Passing
Overhand Passing and Footwork
Overhand Serve

Skills list from chapter 10
Forearm Pass—from serve
Overhand Passing—from underhand pass
Topspin Serve

• *Chapter 11* •

A Method above the Rest
A Question of Quantity versus Quality

If you were to ask me to name only one thing from my training that truly made the difference for me throughout my career, I would, of course, have difficulty answering that question because of how interrelated everything we have been discussing is. However, I did say "have difficulty." If you were really insistent, pushing me to narrow it down, and you prefaced it by saying that you *knew* how important all the other things we have been discussing are, I would have to point to what I am about to teach you in this chapter as that one thing.

Now that you have a solid understanding of what areas and skills you will be working on, and now that you know how to gather the technical information you need, it is time to continue deeper into the process of training. There are two semiopposing ideas or philosophies that help define how a competitor should practice. The terms used to describe these two concepts are *quantity* and *quality*.

QUANTITY

I refer to *quantity* in athletics as a way of training that uses a high number of repetitions. You accomplish this style of training either *by completing a set number of reps*, or *by doing reps for a set amount of time.* The number of repetitions or the set amount of time can vary greatly, depending on what is to be accomplished. The idea here is to repeat a skill enough times so that, over time, the body will naturally learn, improve, and develop the techniques that enhance the performance of that skill. It is through this process that the body starts to build the *muscle memory* needed to perform skills, techniques, and strategies in a relaxed and focused manner. Basically, your body "memorizes" the movements you have performed countless times, and these movements become more *automatic*, thus increasing your chances of executing them well in competitive situations.

Using tennis as our example to demonstrate how we could apply quantity-type training in a sport, say you are an intermediate-level tennis player who wants to improve your serve. Instead of just hitting some serves to each service box without any concern as to whether the serves are in or out or how many serves you hit, you should set a training goal of a certain number of serves that must go into each service box. That number should be fairly high, say around forty or fifty. You should not be concerned, at this point, as to where they land in the box or whether each serve you hit "feels" right—just that you are concentrating generally on good technique and that they go in. Once you hit forty or fifty into each service box, you are through practicing serves for that training session and can move on to other parts of the game.

QUALITY

Training using *quality*, on the other hand, usually includes completing a lower, set number of repetitions in a manner that meets some predetermined quality criterion or standard of performance. *Each repetition of the skill does not count unless it meets the quality standard that's been set.*

It is here, through the quality phase of an athlete's training, that the polish is applied to all movements, mastery becomes a priority, and the body learns to perform without much thought. Training like this allows you to compete in a relaxed manner by merely focusing on a few key points and letting your body repeat what has been so thoroughly performed in practice. (These training concepts of quantity and quality are strongly tied to the development of kinesthetic and proprioceptive awareness discussed in chapter 8, "Separate yet Related.")

Using tennis again to clarify, let's say you want to apply quality-type training to improve your serve. The number of serves you hit would come down to, say, twenty or thirty per service box. However, now you not only have to get those serves *in,* but *must* also accomplish all of these serves with the *right* execution. That means that your grip, ball toss, arm swing, contact point, and follow-through all "feel" so smooth and so good that you know as soon as the ball leaves your racket that it is going into the box. You will come to know that each time you hit a serve like this, it represents exactly the correct technique you have envisioned. It just feels right. Any serve that does not feel this way and/or is not in the correct service box is *not* counted as one of your twenty or thirty correctly executed quality repetitions.

Please keep in mind that these repetition numbers are merely selected to help you understand this principle. You will have to discover for yourself the best numbers to use based on your level of expertise, which sport you play, the skill you are working on, your training goals, and the amount of practice time you have.

FIRST TRAIN QUANTITY, THEN QUALITY

I firmly believe in these strategies for learning, perfecting, and mastering skills and have used them both as a coach and as an athlete. *When starting on a new skill, I found it worked best to apply the principle of quantity.* The more times I practiced on a skill, the faster I learned. (Sometimes the realization of improvement did not occur until a day or two later, but it did occur.) Applying the principle of *quality* is self-defeating at this point because there is no substantial quality criterion that can be set and used for a skill that is either new or has just barely been learned. You do, of course, still practice trying to use correct techniques; you just don't apply the concept of quality as it is so stringently defined above.

However, as you reach a point where you are able to successfully complete many repetitions of a newer skill, and that skill reaches an acceptable level of performance, you can then gradually shift from a concept of quantity to one of quality. Start by setting a smaller number of repetitions (out of the total number of repetitions) that must be completed with a *higher level of execution* than all other attempts or completions of that skill, technique, or strategy.

For example, if you have been used to completing a certain number of repetitions of one skill, say twenty, allocate a certain number of those repetitions to be completed with a higher level of execution (higher standard or level of performance) than the others, like five of those twenty. Complete all your reps, but make sure that the designated smaller number of reps is completed at the level of execution that you have predetermined.

Using basketball free throws to demonstrate this concept, a player may set an objective of making a total of thirty free throws (quantity), with the *quality* goal of also accomplishing this four times in a row with excellent form at some point during the drill. If the player can't do this, then he or she must continue to shoot baskets beyond thirty until four shots in a row have been made with excellent form.

On the other hand, if the player scores four quality free throws in a row before making his or her overall total of thirty, then he or she should continue to shoot until the set objective of thirty has been completed. (Keep in mind it is not the actual numbers in this example that are important, just the principle that needs to be understood. As previously stated, the number of reps you use will depend on the sport, your individual skill level, and what your training goals are.) Choose a number of reps, whether quality or quantity, that will really challenge your ability; however, this number must also be attainable within a reasonable amount of time. This may take some practice and adjustment until you get a good handle on (really understand) your abilities.

THE GRADUAL SHIFT FROM QUANTITY TO QUALITY

As you improve, everything will continue to shift, with the total number of "quantity" reps coming down and the number of "quality" reps going up. Eventually, quality will be the main, and possibly the only, objective you work toward, with you determining the number of acceptable repetitions. When I was training in gymnastics, that number consistently ran to about ten quality repetitions of each skill.

The thing to remember when using the principle of quality during training is that each skill you complete must be performed at a set criterion that you should determine *before* you attempt your reps. Any completed skill that does not meet this standard is not counted. This means that if the total number of quality reps you have chosen is twenty, it may take thirty, forty, fifty, or even more attempts to get in your twenty quality repetitions.

Keep in mind that this progression is a gradual one, and you should not perform quality repetitions to the exclusion of quantity reps until you are ready to work on perfecting or mastering a skill.

Also, no matter which area you are working in (quantity or quality), you will have to be persistent in your efforts. Working on skills using the concept of quantity can get very tedious due to the high number of repetitions, while the concept of quality can be frustrating, depending on the difficulty of the criterion you have set. So make sure the objective for either area is set within your current physical and/or mental limits and stay persistent until the objective or goal is met.

The numbers an athlete sets, whether of quality or quantity, make up what I call the *minigoals* (or *objectives*) of a workout. I refer to these during the description of my own training regimen in high school in Section III. With the skills that fell into the quality portion of this training, my minigoals, I was relentless. I did not leave the gym until they met the standards I had established. (In my opinion, this is another one of those little things that gave me a real edge over my competition.)

Many athletes reading this segment may misconstrue that these two principles of training, quality and quantity, can only be applied to gymnastics. However, *all* sports have fundamentals, technical skills, and/or movements that easily fit this training strategy. Whether you are a football player working on a specific skill like blocking, passing, or catching (or even team-oriented drills as in learning and completing new pass patterns and plays); a tennis player trying to improve your groundstrokes, volleys, or serves; or a volleyball player perfecting your setting, passing, or hitting, applying these two training strategies individually or in combination (just as in the basketball example earlier) increases your chances of mastering the skills and components in your sport.

OVERLOAD IN RELATION TO QUANTITY AND QUALITY REPETITIONS

The word that describes what I was actually doing with many of my gymnastics skills during my own training is *overload*. In this context, the word refers to the practice of skills and movements with such numerous repetitions, and such high levels of execution, that they become internalized both physically and mentally. When you choose to commit yourself to this manner of training, your body "learns" to perform much more instinctively, allowing for more efficient and effective skill production. Basically, every skill or movement you do becomes easier to accomplish, no matter what the situation, and your chances of higher levels of performance during competition increase significantly—especially when the pressure is on. I strongly recommend this form of overload training for any athlete wanting to reach higher levels of performance. (More about the relationship of overload to conditioning later.)

It is, however, important to keep in mind that there is a fine line between overload-type training to attain good execution and *over-training*, which can cause overuse injury or chronic fatigue. One is self-fulfilling while the other is self-defeating. This is where you really have to know yourself and your own physical and mental limits. It is not that you should never push yourself beyond these limits, at times, but just that you need to know when enough is enough and it is time to move on. During tough workouts, you may need to make adjustments in either the quality criteria or the number of repetitions, depending on your physical and/or mental state. Hey—there will always be days when your training is just plain awful, and making adjustments will be both physically and/or mentally necessary.

Striking a balance between knowing when to stop, adjust, or push will be key in staying injury free while still continuing to improve.

You need not look any further than my own sport of gymnastics to find the negative side of overtraining. Elite-level gymnasts, or those seeking elite-level status, have been known to train beyond their physical, and sometimes mental, limits—overtrain. Examples of this abound at the higher levels of gymnastics, where athletes are putting in approximately thirty to forty hours of practice a week, including the likelihood that such athletes at times train with injuries that may not have been given enough time to heal.

However, I want you to keep in mind that it is not necessarily an exact number of hours that should be the limit for everyone (although thirty to forty hours a week *is* a lot), but the amount of practice time your body is capable of handling that determines over- or undertraining. It is just too difficult, if not impossible, to use an *exact* set of limits that fits for all sports and all situations. There are too many variables for this to be appropriate. The physical condition of athletes, their age, the sport they play, the type and number of repetitions they perform, the intensity at which these repetitions are performed, and so on, all play a role. Nonetheless, the following guidelines should be of some help.

If you regularly have to take painkillers to make it through practice, if you have aches and pains that don't seem to go away or which gradually worsen over time, if you are diagnosed with stress fractures—all these may be indications of overuse-type training. Again, it is important to know your own physical and mental limits well enough to be able to make sound judgments on how much to practice. Listen to your body—it will tell you what it needs. Not doing so puts you at risk of short-term injuries like strains, sprains, fractures, and overuse-type injuries as well as long-term, chronic injuries like degenerative joint troubles and/or the spine and disc problems that can plague many elite-level gymnasts.

Also, don't let yourself fall into the trap of telling yourself that unless it hurts, or hurts a *lot*, you aren't making gains. Many athletes like to view themselves as tough and able to withstand a lot of stress and pain. That's not necessarily a bad thing by itself—but if you let that reasoning overrule your common sense about the condition of your body and force yourself to train to real extremes, you are defeating your own purposes by setting yourself up for repeated injuries. That can easily interfere with your ability to progress toward your long-term athletic goals.

Lastly, keep in mind what I discussed about priorities in chapter 4. Yes, your athletic commitments will be right near the top of your priorities list. However, they are not the only commitments you have. Your family and your schoolwork, even some social time, must be important considerations when setting your priorities. This is where striking a balance will be a key component toward helping you stay healthy physically and happy mentally.

TAKING ACTION

Understanding Your Own Quality and Quantity Training

Take out the list of fundamentals and the list of skills and technical elements you developed from the last two chapters.

1. Using the information we have just covered (which you may want to review first), go through both skills lists and mark each skill on it as appropriate for either "quantity" training (it's usually something that you need a lot more work on) or "quality" training (usually something you can already do but would like to perfect).

2. Now go through both lists again. Decide on a number of repetitions for those skills you listed that you feel would fall under the category of "quantity." Write this number down to the left of those skills.

3. Now do the same for skills falling into the category of "quality." However, keep in mind that the number you use here refers to "perfect" completions and is tied to some set of performance criteria you will eventually develop for that item.

   Also keep in mind that the numbers you are writing down for both kinds of skills represent the number of times you will complete that fundamental, skill, or technical element at practice *every day.*

If it seems too difficult at this time to choose a specific number of repetitions for these categories, then just use fifteen or twenty for quantity items and five for quality items. In practical use, you would be able to change these on the spot while training if either number was too few or too many.

4. Once you have finished both lists, put both down in front of you and examine them. What you have just created is the beginning stages of a training/workout program for your sport.

5. **Optional.** If further motivated, you may also want to place a quality criterion to the right of each of the skills you will be practicing with *quality* in mind. Place the heading "Quality Criterion" at the top of this column. Refer again to the chapter if you need to review examples of the types of criteria that can help you focus on quality. (Normally, you will mark quality criteria only for the *quality* items listed; however, it would not hurt at all to write down technical performance hints you need to focus on as you work on the skills falling into the *quantity* category.)

Additionally, after writing down the quality criteria, it is likely you will want to rethink the repetition numbers you have chosen for each item in this category. In a practical sense, these quality criteria will help you determine the actual number of repetitions (of these skills) you will perform.

To further clarify this activity, let's use the short volleyball skills example I created from the "Take Action" activity at the end of chapter 10. Remember that this list was for a more beginning/intermediate level volleyball player, is not meant to be a comprehensive list, and the numbers used are for example purposes only. See Table 11.1.

If you still feel unclear on the information presented after completing the exercise, it would be best that you review this chapter before continuing further with this book. Do not feel inadequate; these are hard concepts for many to understand until they have been through them several times!

Table 11.1 VOLLEYBALL EXAMPLE

	Key:	
	(Q) = Quality (q) = Quantity	

No. Reps/Sets	Fundamentals List from Chapter 9	Quality Criterion
15	Forearm Passing (Q)	- Correct Platform/Contact - Must Be Settable
15	Overhand Passing & Footwork (Q)	- Correct Contact/Position - Must Be Hittable
10	Overhand Serve (Q)	- Full Arm Extension - Correct Contact/ Placement

No. Reps/Sets	Skills List from Chapter 10	Quality Criterion
40	Forearm Pass—from serve (q)	
40	Overhand Passing—from underhand pass (q)	
30	Topspin Serve (q)	

· Chapter 12 ·

An Essential Piece
of the Puzzle

Vital Concepts of Conditioning

$\mathcal{R}$emember the analogy I used in the beginning of this section—
that transforming an athlete into a champion is like building a house?
And how the principles detailed in the first section make up your
foundation—your base of support—and the training process we are
currently discussing is like constructing that house? Well, what do
you think is going to hold all those pieces of your house together?
Here, in chapter 12, I will be giving you the cement, nails, and glue
that not only allow you to assemble your house most effectively but
will also help keep it from falling down.

WHY CONDITIONING?

I know of no athlete, no matter what sport or athletic activity he or
she is involved in, whose performance and skill would not benefit
tremendously from a disciplined and focused conditioning program.
This is not just a little thing, but a "big thing" that will make a huge
difference in improving your ability and performance. It is essential
that you set aside a good block of practice time for this type of training. Neglecting this concept can derail any objectives you may have
set for yourself.

Keep in mind that a workable, appropriate conditioning program can encompass much more than lifting weights. It would

address *all* the physical attributes needed to enhance and improve an individual's performance and ability and decrease the risk of injury. A sound conditioning program would be functional and movement-specific, and it would *not* include unnecessary work that does not enhance an athlete's ability within his or her sport. The program would include, but not be limited to, training for strength, endurance, agility, balance, speed, coordination, power, reaction time, and other such physical capabilities.

There are two main reasons that it is necessary for a competitor to spend some concentrated time on skill-related fitness training, strength training, and conditioning.

First, the stronger, more agile, faster, more powerful, quicker, and more conditioned you are, the better and more consistent your chances are of reaching and sustaining peak levels of execution. It puts so much more of the odds in your favor by putting so much more control over what happens into your own hands.

Second, proper conditioning can greatly decrease the risk of injury. In order for athletes to reach championship form, they need to train hard. This puts a lot of physical stress on the body to the point of fatigue—almost abuse—and it is at this point when you are most vulnerable to injury. The stronger, more conditioned, and better trained you are, the better your body will be able to handle this load.

FUNCTIONAL MOVEMENT-SPECIFIC CONDITIONING NEEDS

When developing a valid, appropriate conditioning program, it is important to consider that each sport, activity, or event you participate in brings with it certain specific training or conditioning needs. Therefore, your conditioning program should consist of functional movement-specific training. This type of training actually conditions *all* appropriate muscles for the sport, as well as trains them in the manner in which they will be used. In addition, it wholly and completely prepares your body for *all* the physical demands placed on it during practice and when competing in your sport.

For example, gymnastics requires muscular strength and endurance, some speed, power, agility, coordination, balance, and quick muscle reaction or response time. However, this sport does not necessitate a great degree of cardiovascular endurance. Wrestling has similar conditioning needs, with more emphasis on cardiovascular and muscular endurance. Team sports like soccer and volleyball require most of the fitness components mentioned above, with different emphasis on upper-body strength, running speed, and lower emphasis on cardiovascular endurance for volleyball. As you can see, you will need to tailor your conditioning program depending on what your sport, or sports, will require from you.

Additionally, if an activity contains a lot of multi-joint-type movements (and most of them do), then a lot of multi-joint-type exercises and/or multi-joint-type weightlifting is used. The specific requirements of the sport dictate how an athlete should train.

To break this down further, almost all athletic movements (in just about any sport) involve a complex and coordinated array of actions between body parts. So whether it is a ballplayer throwing, a boxer punching, a soccer player kicking, a volleyball player spiking, a tennis player serving, or a gymnast swinging to a handstand, *all* of these require a combination of movements involving the legs, torso, and arms to reach their end result. This is why it's essential that any conditioning or training program consist of an approach that accounts for (trains) all involved muscle groups (especially the core—the muscles of the hips/pelvis, buttocks, lower and middle back, sides, and abdominal areas), and, most important, all of them in concert with other muscle groups. That means training all involved muscle groups' ability to function together as one cohesive unit in order to execute the variety of athletic movements required by the sport. This is what makes your conditioning functional and movement-specific.

Let me use a boxer to demonstrate the point made above. It may appear to many watching a boxing match that when a boxer throws a punch (like a jab or right cross), the only body part really involved in this movement is the arm and fist. However, this could not be further from the truth, because what the spectator is seeing is the end result of a sequence of movements starting out with the contact point of the feet on the ground. A boxer's punch is initiated by the muscles in the lower body; this is where the power is generated from. It then moves up into the hips and core of the body, where power is increased by the quickness and strength of these muscles, then up through the chest and shoulder of the punching arm as the arm finally snaps out a fist to complete its task. A well-trained boxer can do this in the blink of an eye. The quickness, strength, and coordination of all of these muscles, bottom to top, formulate the punch that many a novice spectator believes is only in the arm and fist. This same principle can be applied to most physical skills in any sport, justifying how important it is to focus on the body as a whole when training and conditioning.

Also, a well-designed, functional, movement-specific training program will emphasize conditioning your muscles to operate *in the manner in which* they will be used within your sport. For example, if the muscles used in your sport need to be able to perform explosive-type movements, then they should be trained explosively. Quick, agile-type movements would be trained with quickness and agility in mind. And if you require a combination of all of these, then a combination of various types of training and conditioning should be included.

More specifically, if you are a soccer player, it would be very important, as a key part of your training, to use conditioning that requires you to sprint, shuffle, jump, and backpedal quickly, explosively, and at maximum speeds for long and short distances—and to use other forms of strength building and/or resistance training to enhance these movements. It would be a lot less important to run two or three miles at a steady pace (something I have frequently seen soccer players in youth soccer programs doing). On the other hand, if you are a long-distance runner, you should train using long-distance running as one key component of your program, and use other appropriate forms of strength building, resistance training, and/or speed training to enhance your running. You can see how this makes more sense for the long-distance runner than arbitrarily using, for example, the key conditioning movements suitable for soccer players—or any other dissimilar sport.

The specific form of conditioning that you select—such as weight training, calisthenic training, proprioceptive training,

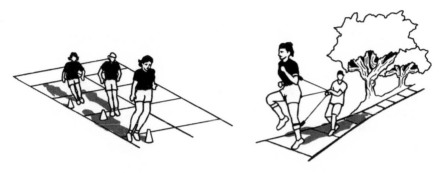

12.1: Conditioning Creates Advantage

resistance training, agility training, speed training, plyometrics,[1] or a combination of these—is pretty much up to you. There are just too many options for any one person to know or list. You can even create your own exercises or conditioning drills, keeping in mind that their sole purpose is to gain *more than enough* strength and ability to perform all the skills of your sport safely, efficiently, effectively, and with ease.

It is also possible to combine a lot of your movement-specific conditioning with the drills you use to improve your skill level, making your training much more time efficient and effective all at the same time. For example, a tennis player could start with his or her racquet on the net, backpedal to hit an overhead smash (that was fed high and deep), then sprint around a cone set off to the side in the alley, then run back to the net. You could repeat this ten times in a row, without stopping, and you will have accomplished both conditioning and skill improvement training all at the same time.

This type of functional, movement-specific training has gained in popularity for all sports in recent times. However, gymnasts have been conditioning in this manner for years. They not only practice their skills repeatedly (and in combination), increasing their level of strength and endurance, but also condition their musculature in a manner specific to how it is used. Dips, plaunches, handstand push-ups, pull-ups, V-ups, L-holds, cross-pulls, etc. (calisthenic-type exercises) are part of many gymnasts' workouts, and all have strong relationships to the movements and skills of gymnastics.

THE EFFECTIVENESS OF FUNCTIONAL, MOVEMENT-SPECIFIC CONDITIONING

My gymnastics training centered on a variety of functional, movement-specific exercises that helped prepare me for still rings competition. However, one specific example really stands out in support of *why* conditioning is so important. In "Putting It All Together—A True Story," Section III, I mention some unique exercises for my shoulders that I designed and carried out to enhance my straight-arm work. The purpose of the exercises was to markedly strengthen the muscles of the shoulder and shoulder girdle, allowing for more efficient and effective movements.

Through this functional conditioning, I not only accomplished my strengthening objective, but also developed my own personal style of movement *and* was able to remain injury free throughout my college gymnastics career. Shoulder pain and shoulder injuries are very common among ringmen due to the amount of pressure placed on the shoulder during practice and competition. It is just the nature of the event—apparently. Yet while others complained of problems in their shoulders, I never had any shoulder injuries during my years of competition, nor did I suffer from the chronic shoulder problems in my twenties and thirties that other gymnasts who worked this event developed—sometimes at an even earlier age. It stands to reason that the extra conditioning and strength training I did for my shoulders had a lot to do with building the strength I needed to perform and also stay healthy. No matter what sport you play, a strong focus on functional, movement-specific conditioning will decrease your risk of injury along with increasing your ability to perform at high levels.

OVERLOAD

The main focus here is to give you some fundamental information about conditioning as it pertains to sports and encourage you to set aside time for this training, as its importance cannot be denied.

As a basic format, you should perform your conditioning exercises using the same *overload* principle that was covered in chapter 11,

"A Method above the Rest." In this context, overload refers to *training muscles beyond their normal workload and to the point of some fatigue, but not to the point of injury*. (More on this point below, in "Basics for Your Conditioning Program.")

Strength and endurance gains are achieved through the use of several sets containing many repetitions and/or increasing the resistance (using resistance bands, increasing weight used, etc.). Both of these basic methods, when done consistently over time, force the muscles to adapt and become stronger and more efficient. From an elementary standpoint, as these adaptations take place and your muscles gain strength and endurance, you then increase the number of repetitions and/or the resistance.

Your main objective with any conditioning program is to give yourself the ability to reach a point of peak muscular efficiency. This means that you will be able to perform the skills and movements in your sport more easily, more efficiently, more effectively, and more safely (with less risk of injury), along with handling all the physical demands of your sport.

The concepts of training described in this chapter can easily be applied to any type of exercise and/or athletic activity. All athletes will benefit from a conditioning program designed for the type of movements used within their own sport, and this is one of the main reasons that functional, movement-specific training has become so popular.

Also keep in mind that there are more conceptually advanced methods for conditioning than the basic overload principle just described. One excellent resource for advanced information regarding these methods is the National Strength and Conditioning Association (NSCA) at nsca-lift.org. I consider this organization to be one of the most credible worldwide authorities on strength and conditioning and encourage you to explore the information available on their website.

BASICS FOR YOUR CONDITIONING PROGRAM

Here are some further basic principles to keep in mind when developing a sound conditioning program. This is not meant to be a comprehensive list, but a list of pointers to help you with your training.

- **Always use good form and technique.** (Quality should always take precedence over quantity in any conditioning program.)
- **Always train equally on both sides of a joint (and all sides of joints with multiple planes of movement), and with *functionality* in mind.** This means you should consider the actual function of that joint. Doing so increases stability of the joint by increasing the strength of the muscles on both (all) sides and the balance between those muscles, along with decreasing the risk of injury.
- **Always train equally on all sides of the body—again, with *functionality* in mind.** Here you want to consider the actual function of the body—how it moves as a unit in relation to the movements that your sport requires and which might occur during participation. This also decreases risk of injury as well as keeps the body in balance.
- **Pay special attention to training the core areas of the body.** They include the muscles of the hips/pelvis, buttocks, lower and middle back, sides, and abdominal areas. Their functional importance and support for *all* physical movements should not be underestimated. They are essential to keeping the body strong and injury free.
- **Perform exercises through the complete and full range of motion.** This increases efficiency of movement and effectiveness of training.
- **Always use spotters or helpers.** Not only do they help with safety, they also can offer encouragement, motivation, help with difficult exercises, and keep your form and technique on track.
- **Never condition beyond the point of diminishing returns.** Whenever overuse injuries become an issue or practice sessions seem to go downhill for no apparent reason, then you should take a look at how, when, and what you are doing for your conditioning. You can defeat the purpose of getting the

most out of your conditioning and can actually *decrease* your strength if you go beyond this point consistently over time.

Basically, what I mean by "never condition beyond the point of diminishing returns" is that you do not want to train to a point where you increase your risk of injury and/or decrease your ability to practice or perform at peak levels. There is a delicate balance here that each athlete may have to find on his or her own. It is also important to keep in mind that practice can be, and *is*, a form of conditioning by itself. Discussing this situation with a good athletic trainer or strength and conditioning coach can help.

- **Endurance training versus strength training.** In general you can train more frequently when doing endurance training because it involves using a steady, lower level of intensity or resistance and a higher number of repetitions than traditional high-intensity, high-resistance strength training. Endurance training is also unlikely to require as much *recuperation* time based on the lower intensity level usually required.

  Additionally, in-season training generally differs a bit from off-season training in that an athlete usually tries to *gain* strength during the off-season, then *maintain* these strength gains during the season (although there are varying philosophies on this point).

- **Make sure to allow time for the body to recuperate between hard training sessions.** Generally, the harder you condition a muscle, the longer it will need to rest in order to recuperate. Most physical educators teach that when you condition a muscle hard you should train using an every-other-day type of approach. So, if you trained your legs hard on Monday you would not train them again until Wednesday. Also, training hard would mean training close to muscle exhaustion, but not necessarily *all the way* to that point. Not following these guidelines can lead to injury and decreases in strength. Just go with the general rule that if you condition a muscle "hard" (yes, this is subjective), then you should give that muscle a good forty-eight hours to rest. You may still use those same muscles during regular practice, but don't condition them "hard" again until forty-eight hours later.

TAKING ACTION

Assessing Conditioning Needs for Your Sport

Part One. For you to train and compete at or near your potential, you must assess the conditioning needs your sport requires. Starting out at a very basic level, I want you to think about the kind of physical movements your body makes when you are playing or practicing your sport or activity:

- What muscles are you using, and *how* are they being used?
- What parts of your body does your sport place the most emphasis on? Is it your legs, your core (back, stomach, and hips), your arms, or are all three areas equally important? (Keep in mind, you will need core work in any sport you train for.)

Your purpose here is to begin creating a *mind-set* for your conditioning. By this I mean you will begin to work out for yourself and understand—and prepare yourself mentally—for the conditioning you will need to do to achieve your potential. At present, there is no need to consider the *type* of exercises you will eventually use (whether it will be calisthenic type, weight training, plyometrics, etc.), just that you start building the foundations from which you will work.

Eventually, when you are ready, you can use this kind of mind-set as a starting point to build your actual conditioning program. This will be a good base for you to begin, and no matter how much conditioning you do or how complicated it becomes, this base should always be a point of reference for you.

Part Two. If you would like to take it one step further, after considering the physical movements of your sport and the parts of your body you use, jot down on paper one or two exercises that work that body part or cause that movement. Try to group exercises in pairs so that you work both sides of the joint, or joints. For example, if you do a push-type exercise with your arms (like a push-up), you would also want to do a pull-type exercise (like a pull-up). Again, the exact type of exercise you decide on at this point does not matter. You are just developing your thinking process for conditioning.

Take a little time to examine the exercises you wrote down. You should be able to identify how making these areas stronger and more efficient will allow you to perform and play at a higher level.

In addition, review "Basics for Your Conditioning Program" above and see if the conditioning exercises you've chosen in this exercise include *all* of these concepts. When you begin to develop your actual conditioning program, you will want to make sure you cover all of these principles.

• Chapter 13 •

Simplifying the Training Process

The Circle of Achievement

$\mathcal{C}$an you think of a time when you worked really hard at something, accomplished what you set out to do, and after a little time had passed you reflected on that accomplishment and something just kind of clicked? I mean, you truly figured out exactly what it was that made your achievement possible?

For me, much of that reflection centered on my sports experiences. It was through this reflection process that I discovered something unique about what had happened to me, or should I say *for* me. As I looked back on the variety of athletic experiences I'd had and focused on the information I gained through all of it, a definite pattern emerged—all the separate elements could be organized into a usable format that I call the "Circle of Achievement" (COA), represented by the COA diagram. The Circle of Achievement can help you better organize the concepts I've discussed in this book, as it gives you four major, related areas to concentrate on in order to achieve your goals. Please refer to figure 13.1 as you read.

The categories of FUNDAMENTALS, ADVANCED SKILLS AND TECHNICAL ELEMENTS, and FITNESS AND CONDITIONING are numbered to assist you in referring to them. The MENTAL AND EMOTIONAL elements are not numbered because the principles encompassed within them are always the same and apply to all areas of athletic endeavor, no matter which sport you participate in. In addition, with these three numbered categories, the

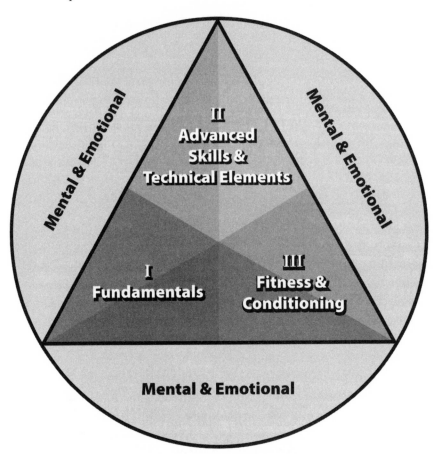

13.1: Circle of Achievement

sport or activity that the athlete chooses to compete and set goals in will govern the exact elements that belong in these areas.

You will certainly notice how *all* of these concepts have been covered in earlier chapters; however, their organization is different in order to simplify everything for you. Your main focus in this chapter should center on this organization, as much of the material itself will take the form of review.

Here is the explanation of each of the parts of the COA, starting with the triangle piece:

COA SECTION I: FUNDAMENTALS

Simply put, fundamentals are

THE BASIC ELEMENTS OR SKILLS THAT AL-LOW THE ATHLETE TO PLAY A SPORT OR ACTIVITY, AS WELL AS EXECUTE THE BA-SIC MOVEMENTS OF ANY SPECIFIC SKILL OR TRICK.

A fundamental can also be a *basic strategic movement* or an actual *basic strategy of the game*. The key here is the word *basic*, for it is what distinguishes this segment of the triangle portion of the Circle of Achievement from the "Advanced Skills and Technical Elements" discussed below. You must place emphasis here because it is the fundamentals that allow the sport, activity, or game to be played at all, much less at a championship level. And it is the fundamental movements of a skill that allow that skill to be performed.

Every sport has these basic fundamentals. In volleyball you must be able to pass and serve as well as shuffle side to side and forward and back. Similarly, in basketball a player must be able to dribble and shoot, along with being able to cut and move to get open. If you cannot perform these skills, you cannot really "play" either game.

Also, any athletic skill has basic components (movements) that allow for that skill to be performed well. These movements are considered fundamental basics for that particular skill. For example, a gymnast could not swing to a handstand very well if he did not have a proficient basic swing. Similarly, a basketball player could not shoot a basketball very well if he or she did not have an excellent follow-through and good balance.

Section I, "Fundamentals," is located in the bottom left corner of the triangle because it forms the backbone for everything developed in Section II, "Advanced Skills and Technical Elements," at the top of the triangle. If you wish to review the material on fundamentals, it is covered in chapter 9, "From the Ground Up."

COA SECTION II: ADVANCED SKILLS
AND TECHNICAL ELEMENTS

In contrast with Section I, "Fundamentals," the segment of Section II, "Advanced Skills and Technical Elements," includes *all elements, skills, movements, and strategies that are not basic in nature.*

These elements comprise the major performance part of the athlete's training. They form the peak, or top of the triangle, because they deserve the athlete's primary focus. They include all the skills, techniques, methods, and concepts needed in order for success to occur. They also include, but are not limited to, all aspects discussed in chapter 10, "Pieces and Parts."

Any skill, technique, method, or concept *beyond* a basic fundamental of your sport is considered *advanced* and would be included in this part of the triangle. However, you should realize that the use of the term *advanced* here is relative to your level of performance. For example, a beginning basketball player might consider shooting a basketball a couple of steps outside the lane (painted area under the basket) as advanced, while a varsity high school player would consider this a fundamental. That same high school player would consider a jump shot several steps outside the lane as more advanced while a professional basketball player may consider this skill a fundamental. So the boundaries of these categories of "Fundamental" and "Advanced" change as the athlete increases in ability.

Additionally, any techniques, methods, and concepts you use to learn, enhance, or improve upon your skill set are included here. Some techniques may include medium- to higher-level strategies that help to fake out your opponent or give you an advantage when you compete—in other words, this section includes all the more complex things you learn when you are becoming "a student of the game."

This Advanced segment definitely overlaps the Fundamentals segment of the triangle, just as there is major overlap between all parts of the triangle. You cannot perform skills well in the Advanced segment if you do not have the fundamentals, strength, and mental preparedness to do so. So all these areas are heavily interrelated and dependent upon each other.

COA SECTION III: FITNESS AND CONDITIONING ELEMENTS

These elements include all the principles, concepts, and strategies surrounding fitness and conditioning-type training. They form the far-right part of the triangle because they help to support and accomplish the Advanced Skills and Technical Elements at the top of the triangle. A complete discussion of Fitness and Conditioning is found in chapter 12, "An Essential Piece of the Puzzle."

COA SECTION IV: MENTAL AND EMOTIONAL ELEMENTS

These elements consist of an athlete's sense of personal responsibility, goals, desire, the CDSPH principle, character and integrity, training and competitive mind-set, support system, and so forth. They include *all* the intrinsic, philosophical, and supportive concepts and principles that comprise a significant part of an athlete's *belief system* (how he or she thinks) and which, in turn, determine how an athlete acts (covered under Section I, "The Principles of a True Champion—Someone Only in Legends?"). In the Circle of Achievement, because of the impact they have on all the other elements, the mental and emotional elements form the circle that encompasses all three points of the triangle.

CIRCLE OF ACHIEVEMENT TRAINING— VOLLEYBALL EXAMPLE

Table 13.1 is an extended example of how you might use the Circle of Achievement to outline your own training strategy. This should help you understand the usability of the COA approach to training. The following model was developed using the sport of volleyball; it would more than likely be used for intermediate-level players. Keep in mind that it is *only* an example and should not be misconstrued to be a comprehensive list of fundamentals, skills, drills, and conditioning for that sport. There most assuredly would be additional and/ or different drills, skills, and exercises placed under the categories of

Table 13.1 TRAINING REGIMEN: VOLLEYBALL

Number of Reps/ Sets or Time	Description	Quality Criterion
I. Fundamentals		
15 minutes	General Warm-up & Stretch	
4 sets	W-Shuffle Drill	Perfect body position, footwork, platform
4 sets	Blocking Steps (1,2,3 step)	Perfect balance, hand placement, penetration
4 sets	Attacking Warm-up	Perfect approach, jump, arm swing
II. Advanced Skills & Technical Elements		
4 sets/20 each	Passing—Miniature Volleyball	10 reps with perfect footwork, contact point, platform
30 reps	Serving	10 to each zone (with emphasis on technique)
20 each position	Service Receive	5 each position with perfect platform, contact point, body position
20 minutes	Setting—to partner	Strong focus on good technique
10–20 reps each	Attacking (each attacking position)	Strong focus on good technique
30–45 minutes	Team Simulation	10–20 kills, blocks, passes, digs—whatever major focus is

III. Fitness & Conditioning

Note: Numbers (column 1) in this section are dependent on the current level of fitness. The Quality Criterion focus (column 3) should be on good technique and form on all exercises.

Agility & Conditioning:

_____	Wind Sprints	Focus on good technique & form
_____	Hills	Focus on good technique & form
_____	Sit-ups	Focus on good technique & form
_____	Ladders	Focus on good technique & form
_____	Push-ups Etc., etc.	Focus on good technique & form
	OR	

Weight Room Strength Training & Plyometric Work:

_____	Squats	Focus on good technique & form
_____	Jump/Press-ups	Focus on good technique & form
_____	Ball Crunches	Focus on good technique & form
_____	Bosu Ball Work	Focus on good technique & form
_____	Back Extensions	Focus on good technique & form
_____	Leg Curls	Focus on good technique & form
_____	Box Jumps	Focus on good technique & form
_____	Bench Presses Etc., etc.	Focus on good technique & form

I. Fundamentals, II. Advanced Skills and Technical Elements, and III. Fitness and Conditioning that are not included here.

The training regimen in table 13.1 is designed for a volleyball *team*; the same principles can be used by any *individual* on that team for the position they play. For example, a defensive player could fill out the Circle of Achievement using only fundamentals, skills, and technical elements and conditioning relative to his or her specific needs and/or playing position.

I must also reemphasize that this training regimen example is not meant to be all-inclusive, nor is it necessarily completely accurate. It is only meant to demonstrate the use of the Circle of Achievement in the breaking down of a sport—in this case, volleyball. Keep in mind that the Circle of Achievement is very adaptable: fundamentals, skills, and technical elements and conditioning components can be added, changed, or removed, depending on your needs. A format like this can be as flexible as you want it.

In addition, it is important for me to point out that none of my own training was ever written out in the same way that this volleyball example is here. It was just the way I practiced, and it wasn't until I had spent time coaching, as well as reflecting on my training, that I realized the format it had taken. I was then able to write it out in an organized manner.

If you are able to write out your training regimen using the Circle of Achievement, it will enable you to really concentrate on what you will need to include and make it a lot less likely that you will forget anything.

CIRCLE OF ACHIEVEMENT TRAINING— GYMNASTICS STILL RINGS EXAMPLE

Following in table 13.2 is a second example of how an athlete could use the Circle of Achievement to develop a training regimen—this time for the gymnastics still rings event. This model was developed, as I remember it, using my own high school gymnastics training as a guide; I used this type of training regimen during the middle of my high school season. Skills were added or removed all year long, depending on changes that needed to be made; again, this type of format can be as flexible as you want.

Because this regimen contains the skills and terminology of the gymnastics still rings, it may be difficult to follow if you are unfamiliar with this sport. It is included here so that you have another example of how the COA can be applied. Do not feel you have to take a lot of time to study the still rings just so you can understand it—it is up to you if you want to do that or not. This breakdown is included here to help give you the idea of how another sport, this time an individual one, can be broken down into a comprehensive and flexible training program using the Circle of Achievement.

As you scan through this regimen, look for the similarities between this regimen and the volleyball team regimen given in the earlier example. The parallels between the two should be easy to identify.

FINAL THOUGHTS ON THE COA

I am firmly convinced that most, if not all, of the principles covered in the Circle of Achievement can be applied to any sport or athletic activity. It is just a matter of your thinking it through, adopting the principles of a true champion as outlined in this book, and then breaking down your sport according to the sections in the Circle of

Table 13.2 TRAINING REGIMEN: GYMNASTICS STILL RINGS EVENT

Number of Reps/ Sets or Time	Description	Quality Criterion
I. Fundamentals		
15 min.	General Warm-up & Stretch	
2–8	Basic Swings	Swing to horizontal or above, both front & back
3	Warm-up Dislocates	Chest & body well above the rings
4–5	Straight Arm Swings to handstand with feet on straps	Fast as possible, freeze at top, no swing
4	Handstands	Solid, no wobble
II. Advanced Skills & Technical Elements		
5	Dislocate Straight-Arm Shoots	Quick, solid, no swing, excellent form
10	Dislocate Straight-Arm Shoots & Straight-Arm Giants	Quick, solid, no swing, excellent form
8–10	Pike Double-back Dismount	Attempts (new skill)
5	Double-back Dismounts	Must land on feet, only one step allowed
2	L-Cross warm-ups	No hold
2	Iron Cross warm-ups	No hold
2	L-hold Press Handstand warm-ups	2 sec. hold
3	Front Halves of a routine	Solid, very little swing, good form, L-Cross held 2–3 counts
3	Last Halves of a routine	Solid press, solid handstand no swing, Iron Cross held 2–3 counts, only one step on dismount
1–2	Full Routines	Quality Criterion same as both front and last halves of a routine.

(Continued)

Table 13.2 (Continued)

III. Fitness & Conditioning

6	Power Dislocates	As high as possible
8	Handstands	Solid, no wobble, perfect form
3 sets of 4	Cross Pull-outs with spotter	Good form, to level, last cross held 2–3 counts
4	Malteses with spotter	Held level with light spot, 2–4 counts each
2 sets of 60	Dips	
2 sets of 10–15	Handstand Push-ups	
2 sets of 10–15	Pull-ups	
4 sets of 5	L-holds	Last one on each set held 3 counts
10	Handstand Push-ups	(Cross Machine Training)
10	Straight-arm Inverted Presses	(Cross Machine Training)
20	Straight-arm Circles in a handstand	Solid as possible (Cross Machine Training)

Achievement. Of course, not everything will fit perfectly. Each sport has too many variables to make that possible. However, the concepts laid out here should all have relevance, no matter what athletic activity you are training for.

Take note also that this framework works equally well with individual sports *and* team sports—as the two training regimen examples demonstrate. The reason it works just as well for both types of sports is this: any member of a team who takes the approach that he or she will work to become the best they can be must follow the same principles as any athlete in an individual sport. The framework outlined in the Circle of Achievement serves as a common thread between all sports and/or athletic activities. It's what binds all athletes together, making them more alike than they are different—because it outlines the path they all must follow in order to achieve championship levels. The differences between sports are really just part of the specific environment you have to consider, contend with, adjust, and adapt to, if you want to achieve any measure of success. In the end, it will be the amount of effort and work you put forth that will make the biggest difference in the accomplishment of the goals you've set. This is true for any sport, individual, or team.

TAKING ACTION

Pictorial Version of Circle of Achievement—Your Sport

Even though the two previous examples given for the Circle of Achievement (volleyball and gymnastics) are very functional and usable, they don't demonstrate how all the principles discussed throughout the book are connected, nor do they address your sport directly. For this purpose, let us work together on developing a very basic and pictorial-type model using your sport as the foundation.

1. Get yourself a sheet of blank paper and draw a circle on it as big as the paper itself. Now draw a triangle in the circle so that each point touches the inside of the circle. It should look roughly like the diagram of the Circle of Achievement, only larger. (See Figure 13.1.)

2. Now, using the three empty spaces formed within the circle but outside the triangle, write the main principles discussed in Section I of this book. Place them in any, or all, of the three spaces you wish. (Several are listed in the first sentence under the subheading "Mental and Emotional Elements" in this chapter.) You can abbreviate them if you like, just so you know what they are.

3. Next, just inside the bottom left corner of the triangle, list three fundamental skills of your sport.

4. At the top of the triangle, list three advanced skills and technical elements of your sport.
    In both of these cases (steps 3 and 4), you can use the fundamentals and skills you listed in the exercises at the end of chapter 9, "From the Ground Up," and chapter 10, "Pieces and

Parts." Or if you wish, develop new ones based on what you learned in this chapter.

5. At the bottom right of the triangle, list three different conditioning exercises that you believe you might use to train and improve your level of performance and physical condition.

6. When you have finished, put the diagram down and take several moments to look it over. Read through what you have placed in each area, and using the knowledge you have gained on the principles and concepts in this book, think about how all of these items support and/or connect in some way to each other. Are you able to see the connections? You may want to draw lines to connect the items where you see these relationships. How about the importance all these concepts have to your success as an athlete? Write this down if you want to keep it for future reference.

Even though the above demonstration is a very basic and incomplete example, it should help to visually clarify how the Circle of Achievement can help organize and simplify your training. The thought process it helps to create in you will become most important when you actually sit down to develop your own "road map" for athletic success. Remember, your thought process is what helps dictate your actions!

· Chapter 14 ·

A Blank Slate to Work With

Circle of Achievement Worksheets

$\mathcal{N}$ow that you have been through two sections of this book, take a closer look at your sport of choice and your own development within that sport (what you are currently doing compared to what needs to be done), using the concepts you have learned and the Circle of Achievement. In order to get you thinking more in depth about your sport and training from this perspective, I have provided a blank set of worksheets you may wish to duplicate and use when applying the Circle of Achievement to your particular sport. These worksheets contain places to fill in the breakdown of your sport in the areas of Fundamentals, Advanced Skills and Technical Elements, and Conditioning. They are more functional and practical than the lists you previously experimented with in the "Taking Action" exercises. There is also a place to write down miscellaneous notes or things you want to remember.

These worksheets can be used as a basic tool to better organize your thoughts and help you get your main ideas down on paper, but you don't *have* to use them. While I did work out all my fundamentals, conditioning, and advanced skills mentally during the time I was competing on the still rings, I never wrote any of it out on paper.

The idea is to use the worksheets if you find it helpful. So, while some of you will want to plot out all your training in detail at least once to figure it all out, in most cases or situations you will use these worksheets to plan just the training elements that are not emphasized enough in your normal practice, those that aren't being trained to your satisfaction, or those that aren't being trained at all. Feel free to copy as many worksheets as you like and use them in any way you see fit.

CIRCLE OF ACHIEVEMENT WORKSHEET
Sport/Activity and Goals

Sport/Activity: _____

Goals: _____

_____

_____

_____

_____

_____

Sport Breakdown: Fundamentals

Time or No. of Reps	Fundamental Skill	Quality Criterion (if any)
_____	_____ →	_____
_____	_____ →	_____
_____	_____ →	_____
_____	_____ →	_____
_____	_____ →	_____
_____	_____ →	_____
_____	_____ →	_____
_____	_____ →	_____
_____	_____ →	_____
_____	_____ →	_____
_____	_____ →	_____
_____	_____ →	_____
_____	_____ →	_____

CIRCLE OF ACHIEVEMENT WORKSHEET

Sport Breakdown:
Advanced Skills & Technical Elements

Time or No. of Reps	Advanced Skill		Quality Criterion (if any)
_____	_____	→	_____
_____	_____	→	_____
_____	_____	→	_____
_____	_____	→	_____
_____	_____	→	_____
_____	_____	→	_____
_____	_____	→	_____
_____	_____	→	_____
_____	_____	→	_____
_____	_____	→	_____
_____	_____	→	_____
_____	_____	→	_____
_____	_____	→	_____

CIRCLE OF ACHIEVEMENT WORKSHEET

Sport Breakdown: Conditioning

Time or No. of Reps	Conditioning Exercise		Quality Criterion (if any)
_____	_____	→	_____
_____	_____	→	_____
_____	_____	→	_____
_____	_____	→	_____
_____	_____	→	_____
_____	_____	→	_____
_____	_____	→	_____
_____	_____	→	_____
_____	_____	→	_____
_____	_____	→	_____
_____	_____	→	_____
_____	_____	→	_____
_____	_____	→	_____

CIRCLE OF ACHIEVEMENT WORKSHEET
Notes & Miscellaneous

Individuality

When individuals base their feelings, opinions, choices, or decisions *only on what others* believe to be true, normal, good, right or wrong, without giving any critical thought to their *real* value, then they themselves forfeit much of their own individuality and in turn join the ranks of mediocrity.

Even though people may think of themselves as individuals making unique decisions when they simply adopt certain behavior demonstrated by their peers, in reality each becomes just another small fish in a big sea of insignificance.

You cannot really realize your full potential as an individual until you can truly say to yourself that what you believe, who you are, and what you will become is directly related to what is deep within your soul. This is where true individuality is born.

Anyone wanting to accomplish this must first be true to themselves. For those who live this idea, outside influences become only minor distractions and one's potential and ability to flourish become limitless.

SECTION III

Putting It All Together—
A True Story

You are about to read the story of my journey from ordinary high school student to gymnastics still rings champion. I recount it in fairly complete detail in order to clearly identify the path I was able to forge that took me from mediocre gymnast to top contender. This story should demonstrate, in a way that words by themselves can't, the ideas we talk about in this book. It will give you a rough sketch—an example—of how advanced skills in a sport can be developed and high levels of performance reached, even against tough odds.

While this section contains a lot of detail specific to the gymnastics still rings event, I have done my best to explain and illustrate the various moves and skills mentioned so that you are able to track with me without getting lost. It is my intention that, rather than concentrating on just the details pertaining to the still rings, you will be able to see beyond the specifics of that sport to work out how you might apply what I did to *your* sport.

Just so you know, during that important year in my life you'll be reading about, I didn't yet know about any of the principles and concepts we've talked about and couldn't have told you myself what I was doing that worked, or why. I just knew I had to work as smart and hard as I possibly could to even stand a small chance of realizing my goals. It was only much later, after becoming a coach and teacher, that I was able to analyze my experiences and come up with these principles so that any athlete could apply them and create his or her own success.

• Chapter 15 •

Mission Impossible

The Goal

$\mathcal{I}$t's simply remarkable how one single moment in a person's life can literally change *everything*. I'm speaking of a point when some event or experience occurs and suddenly the way you think becomes much more narrowly focused and less haphazard. It's almost as if the world comes to a momentary stop, or maybe shifts a little, enabling you to see a direction for yourself that just wasn't visible before. For me, that moment, that shift in my world, came toward the end of my junior year in high school.

It was not something I expected or was entirely prepared for, but who really is? The first three years of my high school life stood pretty much like any other normal teenager's. Like most, I was insecure, very concerned about my appearance, and much more interested in the social things going on around school and on the weekends than in schoolwork or athletics. I even remember telling my father, when he questioned me about my poor classroom performance, that the first three years of high school are not counted in your GPA for college! It's embarrassing, in thinking back on it, to realize that I so readily tried to deceive my father to justify my academic failings.

Sports—in my case gymnastics—was just something I did because I enjoyed it and had a little talent. It certainly was not a high priority on my list. I was average at best and competed for one of the lowest level teams in our high school conference. My favorite

179

event was the still rings. Being able to perform swinging movements while demonstrating power and strength on two wooden rings hung from the ceiling—all while trying to keep the apparatus still—held a special attraction for me. However, as a junior in high school I was not really very good at it. I just thought working this event was a fun thing to do. I never suspected that in the very near future my attitude was going to undergo a drastic change.

It was at the end of my junior year that I made a decision that would alter the direction of my life forever. During the gymnastics conference meet in February, toward the end of our season, I had a chance to see a senior gymnast from Addison Trail High School (in Illinois) compete on the still rings. The memory of this event sticks with me even to this day, as if it had happened yesterday. His name was Tom Ware, and he was good—very good. I remember how smooth and powerful his performance was. He had it all: strength, swing, solid handstands, a good dismount. But it wasn't just what he did that was impressive, but how he did it. Tom could swing forward to an upside-down vertical position (handstand) quickly with very straight arms (referred to as straight-arm work), and when he got to this position he did not wobble and had very little swing. It was as if someone had a rope tied to his ankles and quickly pulled him up to a handstand as he swung through a hanging position. And that was not all. While gripping the rings, Tom could hold his body in a "T" position with feet down and arms straight out from his sides, even with his shoulders (called an iron cross, figure 15.1).

He could also hold his body in a horizontal position, facing downward, with his arms straight by his sides as if he was floating on his stomach in midair (called a maltese, figure 15.2). I had never seen anything like it, not even at the Olympic level. Everything he did seemed so effortless.

That was it! That was what I wanted to do. Everything, for me, changed in an instant and what I wanted became clear. It was as if someone had flipped a switch and in that single moment the light went on for me. Rings were my favorite event, and I wanted to compete on them just like he did, and maybe become even better than he was. I did not give any thought to the fact that the highest score I

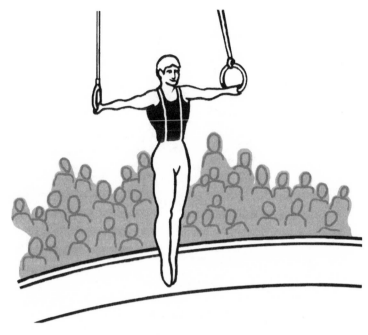

15.1: The Iron Cross

had ever gotten on this event was in the low sixes—and that was only once or twice! I usually scored in the high fives. (In contrast, Tom Ware scored in the low nines.) Nor did I consider that I competed third on one of the worst teams in the conference (I wasn't even the best on our team), while Tom was the best in the conference and would compete for the Illinois High School Association (IHSA) state title on still rings that year.[1] I gave none of this any thought. All that mattered was that I wanted to be as good, or better, than the performance I had just seen.

About a week after the conference meet was our district competition, the first of three competitions that determined qualification to the state finals. It was here that the season ended for most of us. We had a couple of athletes who continued on to the state series in an event or two, but that was it. I was certainly not one of them—not even close!

After this season ended, our head coach passed out a questionnaire that asked what our goals were for the following year—which

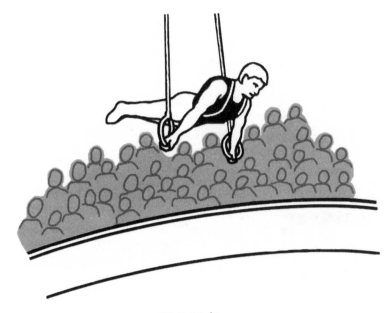

15.2: Maltese

was going to be my final season in high school. Being the assertive teenager that I was, I wrote, "I would like to win the IHSA State Gymnastics Championships on the still rings, score in the nines, and win a full-ride scholarship to compete in gymnastics in college." We were to turn our statements in and meet individually with him to discuss our goals.

This meeting is another event that would stand out vividly in my mind as a pivotal turning point in my life. My meeting took place within a week or two after turning in my form. After reading my goals, my coach did his best to try to explain to me that these were very lofty goals and that maybe I might want to think this through a little more—that maybe these goals were beyond my reach. He wanted me to be "more realistic," as he put it.

I remember thinking to myself that he had no right to tell me what was realistic for me or not—that *I* alone was the one who gets to decide what I think I can accomplish or achieve, not him. I felt misjudged and angry.

Now, I should point out that my head coach was a great guy. He cared about his athletes and was basically concerned that I had bitten off more than I could chew. He knew exactly what level I was at and what level I would need to achieve to accomplish these goals, and he knew I was nowhere near it. He also knew I had never even been close to placing respectably in the conference meet, let alone qualifying out of the district meet into sectional or state competitions—yet I wasn't just talking about possibly making it to the state meet. I wanted to win the whole damn thing on the still rings event. A gymnast can work hard all four years of high school, go to camps, practice at a club, and still not achieve what I was attempting to do—and time for me was very short. I only had nine months until the start of the next gymnastics season. In the same circumstance, if I were the head coach, I would probably have said the same thing to one of my own athletes. (It is part of a coach's responsibility to do this.)

You see, not only was my goal unrealistic, I also had to compete against many athletes who had already participated and placed at the state meet the year before, including then-current Junior Olympic National Champion (and future Olympic Gold Medalist) Bart Conner.

As I look back on this, it becomes important to reiterate how unachievable this goal seemed within the time frame I had. Let me see—even though I had mostly scored in the fives, with a few low sixes thus far, I wanted to win a state championship, score in the nines, and receive a full-ride scholarship in just under a year. That pretty much looked impossible. If I were to try to draw a simple analogy to this using another sport such as football as my example, it would be similar to a second- or third-string quarterback on the worst team in a conference expecting to become the very best quarterback in his state in under a year! Unattainable, right? My friends had the same take on it and found it laughable—something they made painfully clear.

But all of this opposition just bolstered my determination and helped it develop into a very deep desire to prove to everyone, including myself, that I could achieve what I wanted and that they were wrong. (Recall how various kinds of adversity, including the type of ridicule and opposition that I received, can provide an athlete with strong motivation to succeed.) Little did I know what I was setting myself up for. I really had no clue, at the time, of the amount of work that would have to go into the accomplishment of a goal like this.

BREAKING IT DOWN

One of the first decisions I made was to sign up for gymnastics camp, as I had the previous summer. There I could work with some of the best coaches and gymnasts in the country. My father said he would pay for half if I did the same. I really wanted to go to camp, so paying half was fine with me. The first summer I had gone, I really had had no objective other than to go to camp, do gymnastics, and have fun—and not necessarily in that order!

This time my attitude would have to be different. I was going for the specific purpose of accomplishing something. I knew that the social aspects and fun that normally occur as part of a camp experience would most assuredly have to take a backseat to why I was there. (Hmm . . . looks like I was learning something!) The camp wouldn't begin until later in the summer, but I knew that I needed to get to work right away because I was so far behind. This fact prompted me to join a gymnastics club called Gym Forum. It was there that my training really started. Joining this club and going to camp were two choices I made that helped put me on the right path.

There was no men's gymnastics coach at the club, just the facilities to use and a women's coach. This made things a little more difficult, since the responsibility for setting up my workout, as well as how and what I was going to work on, fell completely on my shoulders—there was no one else. Don Carney, the women's coach, was a great spotter and could give me assistance (a "spot") on some tricks I was unable to do by myself, but the decisions about what I should actually be doing and how skills should be performed were entirely my responsibility. As a women's coach, Don did not know a lot about the still rings event.

I used the knowledge gained during the previous summer's camp experience to start teaching myself the tricks, skills, and techniques I thought I needed. I did have one major plus on my side, however. My younger brother was also a gymnast at the time, and, since we worked out together at the club regularly, he became my "assistant" coach. He was a tremendous help to me throughout high school and college.

The still rings event consists of many different types of skills. These skills are put together in order to form a routine (combination of tricks) that a gymnast performs in competition and then receives a score for. In order to simplify my training on these skills, I decided to break the entire still rings event down into three types of movements or skills.

First, there were swing moves. I wanted to perform them just like Tom Ware, with straight arms and solid as a nail (no wobble or unnecessary movement). Any good high school ringman could swing to a handstand, but only the very best could do it with straight arms (called "straight-arm" work). Swing movements allow a ringman to show off his style and control. The faster, more explosively, and more solidly these skills are executed, the more impressive straight-arm work becomes (figure 15.3).

The next category centered on the strength part of the event. For me, that meant an iron cross (figure 15.1) and/or a maltese (figure 15.2).

Both of these skills take a tremendous amount of strength, and the way a gymnast performs them can make all the difference in the world. Tom Ware influenced me in this area as well. He did a cross better than anyone I had ever seen. (In fact, it was *how* he did his swing moves and strength moves that set him apart from everyone else.)

The last category of skills I would concentrate on was the dismount. This was the finishing portion of a gymnast's routine and represents the exclamation point of the performance—a dramatic and exciting combination of moves. My dismount of choice was a "tucked double-back." This skill is accomplished by performing two summersaults in midair in a balled-up (tucked) position once you have released the rings (figure 15.4). The key on this or any

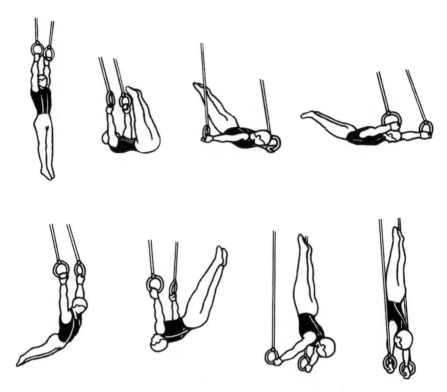

15.3: Forward Straight-Arm Shoot to Handstand

dismount is to land on your feet while taking the fewest number of steps possible—the best number being zero (called a "stick" because it looks like your feet are "sticking" in place with no movement after you land).

How close was I to any of these skills as I started? Not very! I could swing to a handstand but with very bent arms, and bent legs, and I was pretty wobbly when I got there. I even fell out of the handstand regularly during practice. You had to hold this position the required two seconds for a judge to give you credit for it. And my cross was terrible—so bad that I'm not sure you could call it a cross. It was more of an elevator going down! For me to hold it, or in my case hesitate in the position momentarily, I had to bend my arms and wrists and stop above the level "T" position. If I did not do this, it was "elevator city," and I would just fall through in slow

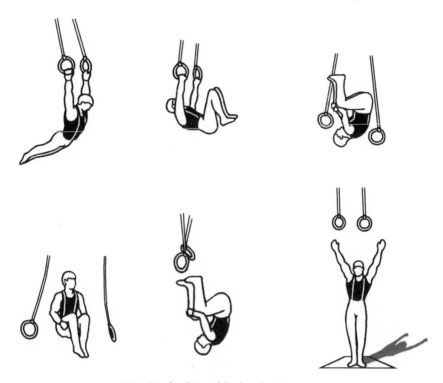

15.4: Tucked Double-back Dismount

motion. Boy, was it an ugly iron cross. And my maltese at the time isn't even worth mentioning—I was much further from a maltese than I was from a cross. I neither had the strength nor technical ability to achieve this level of skill performance, and "realistically," I was much more than a year from gaining these abilities! Well, enough said.

The skill I was probably closest to achieving was the dismount. A double-back was not that difficult to accomplish. The hard part was landing solid on my feet. This, of course, was going to take work. My brother's help became very important to me here. Since I did not have a coach to help with technique, it was my brother who would critique my skills and give me feedback on how they looked. He was as critical as I was and had a good understanding of what I wanted to accomplish.

• *Chapter 16* •

Take a Walk in My Shoes

Club Training and Camp

$\mathcal{S}$o now I had decided what I wanted to do and how I wanted these skills to look. However, I really had no idea, and I mean *no* idea, how difficult this was going to be! I trained at the club after school for three to four hours a day and went there six days a week through the end of the school year.

These early workout sessions were at times very frustrating for me. I would repeat skills over and over again, not seeming to gain any ground or make any improvement for weeks. However, giving up was not an option. Doing so would have meant that everyone was right about my inability to achieve my goals. So it was through these efforts that I started developing a strong sense of perseverance and a concept of *where* the control over one's destiny really lies—it lay only with myself, and no one else. This perseverance, as it turned out, would be severely tested a number of times during the next year.

I continued this workout schedule into the summer, when I replaced school with a job. (I still had to earn half the money to pay for gymnastics camp.) Gymnastics and work became my two most important priorities, while my social life took a backseat. Now, I was never a big partier and I chose not to drink, which had already kind of made me an outcast anyway. Additionally, I was short—not a good thing for a guy's social life in high school. (At the time, I did not realize that the reason I chose not to party and drink was the same reason that I chose to work so hard toward something that did not seem achievable. I was just not going to allow others to dictate what I was going to do.)

Don't get me wrong, I loved going out with friends on Friday and Saturday, going to parties, dances, sporting events, and hanging out at McDonald's (which was our big high school hangout). It was just that those things started to hold less importance for me in comparison with what I was trying to accomplish. I still went out a lot and had great times. I just balanced my life differently from most teens by putting my training at the top of my priority list.

As a matter of fact, I cannot emphasize this idea strongly enough. Many of you reading through this section on my training may misconstrue what I've just said, but I want to make sure you know that I did *not* eat, breathe, and sleep gymnastics. When I was in the gym, I did give 100 percent, both mentally and physically, to my training, but whatever happened in the gym pretty much stayed in the gym. How and what I was going to practice was thought out on the way to or from the gym, or in the gym after I arrived. I only remember a handful of occasions during my senior-year training where I brought practice home with me. Later, I'll tell how one of these occasions had a positive and profound effect on my attitude.

Training, for me, was very focused and intense. It also had its ups and downs—mostly downs in the beginning. Just as I seemed to be improving, I would hit a plateau that I couldn't seem to get past. When this happened I would concentrate more on both the technical execution of what I was attempting and on my physical conditioning, trying to gain the muscular strength needed to accomplish the skill or skills I was working on.

To enhance my conditioning, I developed a unique set of exercises designed to enhance and strengthen the muscles of the shoulder girdle—the musculature responsible for straight-arm work. Straight-arm work was an essential part of any good ringman's routine. I did these exercises religiously every day at the end of practice during my conditioning sessions, all year long. (In college, I was even known to bring ten-pound weights to competitions—something my college teammates thought was hilarious—in order to maintain my shoulder strength.) It was and still is my belief that these exercises were a principal factor in the development of the style of straight-arm work I did on the rings. And straight-arm work eventually became my forte—my strong point. So my training proceeded at a consistent pace of three to four hours a day, six days a week, accompanied by the normal ups, downs, and plateaus that occur with all athletes as they strive to improve their abilities.

It would have been nice if my improvement had continued, even if slowly, throughout the summer; however, that was not the case. I think it was some time around the end of June when it happened. I really hit a wall. Nothing I was working on seemed to get any better. I did not know whether it was a physical or emotional wall—maybe both—all I knew was that time was running short and I was nowhere near where I needed to be. It was less than two months before camp and only about five months before the high school season. Even though I had improved in some ways, I still had a long way to go, and I was running out of time.

I am not really sure what brought about these feelings—whether it had been seeing others competing on television or working out in the gym, or just remembering what I saw in Tom Ware during the past season—but I came to a sudden awareness of how far behind I was. What I do remember is coming home emotionally distraught after a rough practice session one night and sitting down at the table with my father and telling him that everyone was right. I had bitten off more than I could chew, and it did not look as if I was going to accomplish the goals I had set. I was just too far behind and not good enough. I remember him listening intently and looking straight at me, like he could see right inside me. Then, with a very confident pat on the back, he said, "Kirk, you can accomplish anything you set your mind to." I remember thinking to myself that my dad just did not get it.

Ever get that feeling after telling your parents (or friends) something? That they just didn't seem to have a clue about what you were saying? Well, that was the feeling I got after first trying to explain my predicament to my father.

I tried to further clarify how far behind I was, detailing more specifically what I could and could not do, and that I was "light years" away from where I needed to be. But he just repeated his statement with even more confidence and conviction than he had used the first time. In retrospect, I know that he got it perfectly.

My response was, "Do you really think so?" He said, "Yes I do."

That was it. That was all it took. He was my father, and I trusted what he told me. He had always been honest and straight with me, so I believed him, and in turn, I started to really believe in myself. And this belief began to permeate much deeper within me.

I think it was right after this emotional conversation I had with my father that an important shift in my perception took place. Instead of looking at how far I was from my goals, which was pretty far, I started focusing much more on improvements I had on a daily basis. Basically, I started trying to improve each and every day, taking pride in any and every improvement I made, no matter how small.

From that point forward, I found my summer workouts had a lot more peaks than valleys. Skills started to develop. My brother saw major improvements—and not only in the technical aspects of the skills I was working on but also in my attitude and confidence. My straight-arm work really started coming along, my strength was improving, and my dismount became easy to do. Things were looking up, and camp was just around the corner.

CAMP

The gymnastics camp I attended was called Tsukara Gymnastics Camp, and it was located in Hayward, Wisconsin, an eight-hour drive from where I lived. I felt really good about going this time because I had improved so much over the previous summer. By the time I left for camp, I was actually doing some pretty good swing work, starting to hold my cross and only taking one or two steps on my double-back dismount. In fact, I had improved to the point where I was probably one of the better ringmen at Tsukara.

If my memory serves me right, it was during camp (or not long before it) that I started to set smaller individual objectives, or what might be called minigoals, for each skill I was working on. Before this, when training at the club, I had just worked on three categories: swing (straight-arm work), strength (crosses, malteses, etc.), and my dismount component (tucked double-back), and I had done it in a fairly random fashion. I would do many repetitions of one of the above skills, or group of skills. I would make some, miss some, and then move on to the next movement or skill. I had really grown, both physically and mentally, over the last four or five months, and I was now at a point where I was completing many tricks 95 to 100 percent of the time. Of course, their execution was not perfect, but I was finishing them.

However, since gymnastics was a sport of perfection, I now felt the need to move from a framework of *quantity* (encompassing a lot of repetition before moving on to practice another skill) to a framework of *quality* (encompassing set criteria of performance for each skill that must be achieved before moving on).

I began setting specific objectives for every component I was working on. I set several minigoals that I would complete each practice session:

- ten perfect straight-arm shoots to handstand;

- ten bent-arm reverse or back giant swings to a handstand (from a handstand, falling backward through a hanging position and back up to a handstand);

- eight to ten straight-arm shoots to a handstand and reverse giant swings to a handstand in combination;

- three sets of three crosses and cross pullouts using a helper (pullouts are done from the cross "T" position by pushing down on the rings with your hands, keeping arms straight, until you are in a support position);

- four malteses with a helper; and

- five double-back dismounts to my feet.

I also set minigoals of quality regarding other requirements and skills I was working to master and continued using the quantity criteria for tricks I had left to learn. Some of these I added to the conditioning part of my training, while others I interspersed throughout my workout.

It is very important to point out that the number of quality repetitions I set for each objective did not consist merely of executing a set number of completions. I began to develop specific quality criteria for every skill, and I had to accomplish these criteria each and every time I performed that skill. It wasn't just that I did these numbers, but *how* I did each one that mattered most. If I did a skill and it did not meet the performance criteria I had set for that skill, it did not count. For example, my straight-arm work had to explode (meaning to move with suddenly increased speed instead of maintaining a steady pace) as I swung through a hanging position right to the handstand, and when I hit the handstand, I would not accept any movement (wobble) in my body. It had to be solid as a rock. Because of this, it could take twenty or thirty attempts, sometimes more, before I reached my goal of ten quality repetitions.

I applied this philosophy to everything I did on the still rings. IF IT WAS NOT GOOD ENOUGH, IT DID NOT COUNT. Anything less was unacceptable. This made my workouts long. I would repeat things until I got them right, and my definition of "right" would change over time. As I got better and could meet my objective more easily, I would increase my expectation of how well I wanted to perform the skill.

I kept this attitude throughout high school and throughout my career. I just would not accept anything less. You can imagine that when I had a bad day, it was *really* a bad day! I can remember, even at camp, days where everybody would be gone and I would not leave until I had met my expectation.

Once I had completed my swing work and dismount work, I would then concentrate on my strength components. This included crosses and malteses along with a variety of other required tricks and skills, conditioning, and my own unique exercises for my shoulders. The strength component alone took about an hour and would always be done at the end of practice when I was the most tired.

I used this type of training regimen throughout the summer and through my senior year. The big difference between my practices before camp and those I executed after camp was that I had mostly emphasized quantity before my camp experience and changed to emphasize quality during and after camp. This is because my initial learning phase was ending while my perfecting phase was just beginning; in order to continue moving my level of performance up, I found it necessary to make this change. Hard? Yes. Worthwhile? Definitely. These practice routines were a major aspect of my training that I believe helped me gain on my competition. And I am sure some people thought I was nuts!

Camp, which started as a place for me to learn and develop new skills, became a place to test these skills against other gymnasts from other states. Also, I was starting to be noticed by the athletes and coaches in the camp. This was a good thing because I wanted to compete at the college level and some of the athletes were college gymnasts training for the summer, while some of the coaches had college contacts if they weren't college coaches themselves. I took pride in this, and it motivated me to continue to work hard. It was of great benefit to train with some of the best high school and college gymnasts and coaches in the country, and I picked up additional technical information that I would use later in the year as I continued to improve.

At camp, we trained in the morning, afternoon, and some in the evening. There were afternoon activities and breaks where we could go water skiing, sit on the beach, or play table tennis, as well as evening activities where we could socialize. The camp counselors took us out to the movies one night as well as held a big dance toward the end of our stay. Oh, did I forget to mention it? Tsukara was coed! I just loved my experience there—not only was it a great place for me to train and learn, but it also helped me to grow as a person. I would highly recommend a sports camp to all athletes who want to improve their abilities.

Chapter 17

Putting It to the Test

Senior Year

$\mathcal{A}$fter returning home from camp, I went back to the club to train and continued using the principles and strategies I had developed over the previous six months to improve my skills. The summer was over, my camp experience had been very rewarding and enjoyable, and school was about to start. I did not hold down a job during the school year—there was no time. I just went to school, did homework, and worked out at the gym. My training took the same format that it had toward the end of my junior year in high school—I spent three to four hours a day at the club, six days a week. I kept that workout schedule the same until the high school gymnastics season began.

My straight-arm work had really come along and continued to improve. However, I was only able to accomplish it swinging forward, but not backward. (At the time, I thought it was imperative that I was able to swing with straight arms in both directions. I would learn later that this was not the case.) I was also still having problems doing a maltese and pulling out of my cross, but the cross by itself was very strong—so strong, in fact, that I was planning to use two of them in my routine this season. One would be an L-cross pullout, which I hoped to pick up soon (figure 17.1). I thought, hey—why not? Even though I had had difficulties during the beginning and middle stages of my training, and there were still skills I needed to learn, almost everything else seemed to be improving and

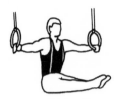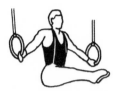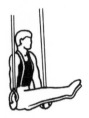

17.1: The L-Cross Pull Out

coming together fairly well and I saw no reason why that would not continue.

Of course, planning to do something and actually doing it are two completely different things. This concept I had yet to discover! My press to handstand, the handstand itself, and my tucked double-back dismount were all pretty much ready to go. At this point, three months before season, things looked good, and I could not wait to show my coach what I had learned in such a short time and to test myself against other gymnasts in actual competition. Just three months until tryouts.

These first three months of school went fast. Tryouts came, and my coach and teammates were impressed. They could not believe how far I had come in such a short time. This reaction was very rewarding for me and helped build my confidence level. But little did I know that this confidence was about to be tested—and would continue to be tested throughout the season. There was still the matter of straight-arm work in reverse, cross pullouts, and a maltese. None of these skills were coming easily. It was now three months into the school year, and I was no closer to mastering any of them than I had been at the end of camp—especially the reverse straight-arms. I could swing backward to a handstand with bent arms, but that was it. There seemed to be a gap forming between the skills I had already learned, as they continued to improve, and those I had yet to learn. This would be something I would have to address before I started competing.

As soon as the high school season started, it became immediately apparent that my training schedule would have to change. Our high school practice was only three hours long, and I was working not only the rings, but also the all-around position for my team—which included performing four other gymnastic events! (My summer training did include work in the all-around, but my passion and majority of time was spent on the still rings.)

I knew that, as important as my goals were to me, it was not all about "me," and, as a senior member and captain of the team, I rightfully felt the weight of this responsibility. The team had to come first.

However, the extra time I spent on the other four events fulfilling my team commitment made it impossible for me to get in the amount of practice that I felt I needed on the rings, as I was definitely still behind in several areas. My expectations on the skills I had already learned had increased tremendously (I was at the point of trying to really perfect these skills), and my conditioning had become very focused and extensive. But there was just not enough time in a three-hour practice to accomplish what I wanted—and my coach had to leave at 6:00 p.m. He had a family to raise and couldn't stay any later.

As a result, I started practicing at night at the club I attended during the summer. I would practice from 3:00 to 6:00 at school, quickly run home to eat dinner, then head to the gym to practice from about 6:45 to 8:30 or 9:00. This I did almost every day during the week, and on Saturdays I also went to the club for a couple of hours in the afternoon after my high school team practice. So my in-season training consisted of approximately four to five hours of practice a day, six days a week. If there was something I wanted to do socially, like go to a game, a dance, or something else (usually on Friday nights), I would stay at school after my teammates left to finish my conditioning, instead of going to the private gym. I can't even begin to count the number of times I would still be training while students were starting to pile into the main gym of our high school to watch a basketball game.

When I finished, and only when I finished, did I go home, shower, and go out. What I wanted to accomplish in gymnastics was my number-one priority, and everything social became secondary. Some might ask, "What fun was there in that?" Realistically, I only missed about an hour or so on Friday nights compared to other kids, and most athletic events didn't start until around 7:00. My curfew was midnight, so I had plenty of time to go out. Many of my friends were just watching television during this time frame, and all the extra practice I put in during the week was never really an issue. Everyone I knew went out only on the weekends. But even if this had not been the case, it would not have mattered. My greatest enjoyment would eventually come from being able to perform skills much better than others could—not from the time I was missing going out! There is no reward comparable to the inner satisfaction gained from accomplishing what you want through sweat and hard work.

I firmly believed that the decision I made to work out at a gym after my high school practices was essential to the achievement of my goals. However, it was this same decision that almost derailed my plans and put me at risk of a possible athletic suspension. In the 1970s, when I was competing, the IHSA (Illinois High School Association) had a rule that would not allow an athlete to train *for* a club team during their high school season. What I was doing could be interpreted as a violation, but I was unaware of this rule until a girl from my high school, who trained at a gymnastics club, reported my extra practice to our athletic director. I am not sure exactly why she did this, other than she had been told not to train at the club during the season and felt that what I was doing was unfair. I could think of no other reason.

The athletic director pulled me into his office and explained that what I was doing broke the IHSA guidelines for athletics in Illinois. (The premise behind this rule was to keep athletes from being trained by their club coach during their high school season, giving them an unfair advantage.)

I replied that our high school practices were not long enough for the type of training I needed to accomplish what I wanted. I also explained that I was not being trained by anyone but myself and was only using the facility as a place to work out and not getting any extra coaching.

We respectfully went back and forth regarding this issue until he finally said that there was nothing he could do about it and if I got caught training there again I could be suspended and would then be unable to compete for my high school team.

This put me in a terrible quandary, for two reasons. First, I believed I had good character, and for me to continue to do something that went against my athletic director's interpretation of this regulation didn't sit well. But second, if I stopped my after-school training, there would be no way I would accomplish the goals I had set. Yet if I continued and got caught, the outcome would be the same.

Even though I did not like breaking a rule (or in this case an interpretation of a rule), I was not seeking an advantage anyone else couldn't also get through longer workouts in their own gym, not hurting myself or anyone else, and not being trained by anyone outside the school (even though there was no proof of this other than my word). I simply did not consider what I was doing as any form of "cheating." To me, it was not any different than if an individual went to the local YMCA after their regular high school practice and did extra weight lifting to improve their strength, and thus their abilities. It seemed strange to me that the weight-lifting activity would have been fine while what I was doing was not.

If I wanted to achieve my goals, I really had only one option that seemed reasonable—I chose to continue my self-training at the club. Because I was not actually receiving club training by an outside coach, what I was doing did not really violate the letter of the rule, and I felt the athletic director's interpretation of the rule was therefore incorrect. I felt that I had not come this far to allow something or someone else to arbitrarily cut off my chances for success. I would not have been true to myself if I made any other choice, so I chose to continue.

With the season underway, the first competition was just around the corner. I had only about three weeks of practice left before my first ring routine would be put to the test. It became apparent fairly quickly that I would have to make some adaptations in the strength area of my original routine. I was still unable to do a maltese and a cross pullout, so I made a couple of adjustments and continued preparing for my first meet. I figured I could add these two skills later on in the season. (In hindsight, I am sure that most athletes need to make adjustments along the way; however, this was difficult for me to understand at the time. I had spent about nine months working on them and was still having trouble.)

As it turned out, changing the strength combinations was not a big deal. I just performed an L-cross (a cross with your legs lifted up and straight, parallel to the floor) in the middle part of my routine and a normal cross at the end, right before the dismount. The biggest problem I still had was in the swing portion of my routine. I started my performance by swinging forward to a handstand with straight arms (straight-arm shoot) and then backward to a handstand with bent arms in what is called a reverse giant. But these two moves just didn't look right done together the way I was performing them. There was no deduction for this; just that one skill was being executed at a much higher level than the other. I really couldn't think of any other option at this point, so I kept these two moves in my routine.

My first competitions went well. If I recall correctly, I scored somewhere in the high sevens. This was a two-point increase from the year before, and it was still the beginning of the season. In a sport like gymnastics, where you can win or lose by tenths or even hundredths of a point, a two-point increase was huge. I figured I had "only a little more than a point to go." (I didn't realize at the time that once you start scoring in the eights, every two or three tenths was almost a different level of performance. And in the nines, every one or two tenths was a different level.)

I continued with my training. I was consistent, committed, dedicated, and focused on trying to improve and perfect my skill level. But even with this hell-bent determination, I still hit a plateau similar to those I'd encountered in the earlier part of the summer. I could not seem to improve on the bent-arm reverse giant I was using or do the two strength moves that I thought I needed. No matter how much time I spent on them, I could not seem to gain any more ground. (Looking back now, I know that physically, I was not mature enough to develop the muscular strength and technique needed to accomplish what I wanted—something I didn't realize at the time.) These skills did improve, but they were nowhere near good enough to score in the nines, which is what I would have to do to win the state meet and get a scholarship. So I continued performing my routine with the two crosses and that bent-arm reverse giant.

After several competitions during the first month or so of the season, I was still scoring in the low to middle eights. Even though I was improving, it was not coming fast enough, and it showed in my scores. What had changed from an impossible task at the end of last season to a "just might be possible" task at the beginning of this season was starting to look impossible again.

About midseason, I talked with my coach regarding my frustrations. He discussed these concerns with several good judges and got a handle on why I was not scoring higher. With the addition of this information, it did not take us long to come up with another option that he thought might work. We decided to get rid of my reverse giant swing to a handstand (I just could not execute this skill with straight arms) and try a forward straight-arm giant instead (figure 17.2).

I had never tried this, even during camp, and was unsure how difficult it might be to learn. All I knew was that I would not accomplish my goal if I continued performing my routine in its current form. To my amazement, the forward straight-arm giant was pretty easy—even easier than what I was currently doing—and it looked ten times better.

This was probably because the first skill I performed, the straight-arm shoot, was identical to the giant except the giant added more swing. A shoot to handstand starts at a much lower angle of trajectory than a giant, decreasing the amount of swing and/or power available. The increase in swing with the giant occurred because it is done from a handstand back to a handstand. However, it is because of this extra swing that a giant is almost always harder to control.

I was gratified that this did not seem to be an issue for me. I believe this was a result of all the straight-arm shoot/swing work I had been accomplishing as minigoals during normal training and because of the unique shoulder-strengthening exercises I had developed for this purpose. So I added the forward straight-arm giant to my routine and got rid of my bent-arm back giant. My first two skills now complemented each other well, and both were performed at the same level of execution—at a much higher level than my previous execution.

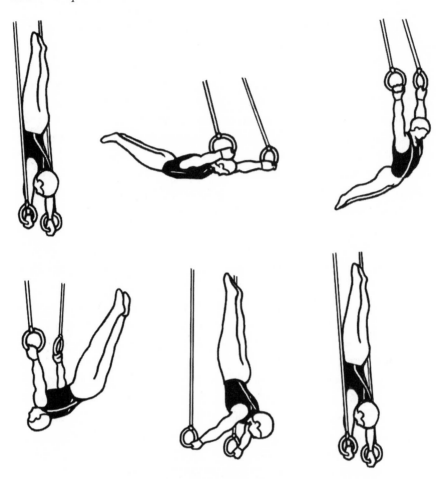

17.2: Forward Straight-Arm Giant

My coach and I also spent some time discussing my planned strength combination. We both agreed that it was best to give up on the idea of using a maltese and cross pullout in my routine and keep the skills I was currently using, at least for high school. I did, however, continue to work on malteses and cross pullouts in my conditioning, with the idea that I would be able to use them in college. Also, continued practice on these would only make me stronger and improve my performance.

Once these decisions and changes had been made, it did not take long before my skills started to flow. It was as if all the pieces of a puzzle were now starting to fit together. I added the straight-arm giant to my minigoals portion of my workout (removing the reverse giant) and practiced all combinations as much as I could in order to perfect them before my next competition.

With my new routine and only about six to eight weeks left in the season, I regained much of my confidence. The routine itself actually took less effort to do, and it certainly looked a lot better—and it had a higher scoring value from a judging standpoint. As always, my brother was a tremendous help to me in this part of my training. He and I would discuss the little nuances that made my routine look its best, especially with the swinging components.

One key to a good still ring performance centers on keeping the rings themselves from swinging while your body swings around them. This is very difficult to do since the rings are not stationary. The faster and more powerful your swinging movements, and the more solidly you can stop in a handstand, the better your performance looks. It was through this process I started to learn how important the little things were. It would be those fine points in a performance that would separate the good from the best, once an athlete has tackled and mastered the major components or skills he or she needs to perform at any given level. This concept would eventually develop into another very important part of my philosophy on training.

I am not sure exactly when it happened, but not too long after I changed my routine, I started scoring above the middle and up into the higher eights. This was a great feeling. I cannot count the number of times before this I had raised my hand to compete, gotten the nod from the judge to go, performed my routine well, and still did not break 8.5. How frustrating that had become! I had put in a lot of time and effort only to have my hopes dashed when I saw my score.

But all of a sudden, my scores jumped close to half a point. The changes I had made in my routine made a big difference, and my efforts looked as if they might really be paying off. I was earning the respect of my friends, my coach, and my teammates, as well as the respect of other coaches and gymnasts around the state. In a sport like gymnastics, where the scoring system brings with it great subjectivity, sometimes the fact that people know you and respect who you are is as important as what you do. I had come a long way and was not about to stop here!

However, adversity would rear its ugly head again in the not-so-distant future.

As the season progressed and competitions intensified, I continued to score in the high eights. The end of the season and the state series were drawing near, but I had yet to break a nine. My routine was beginning to look polished, but my scores did not reflect this. I remember one instance where I had completed what I thought to be a very good performance worthy of a 9.1. However, when the scores came up, one judge had me in the low nines while the other flashed a middle six. That was almost a three-point difference, and the two judges had to confer and adjust both scores due to the large discrepancy. I just about fainted. I wondered how that could even be possible. Two certified judges looking at the same performance using the same criteria, yet their scores came up well over two points apart. Unbelievable.

I grew to realize that even though I had complete control over how hard I worked, what I would accept from myself, the goals I set and the process I used to try to accomplish them, I certainly did not have full control over my final score. That would be left up to someone else—a stranger, a judge—someone sitting in a chair who watched what I did and made a decision based on a set of subjective criteria. This I did not like, but it only fueled the desire I already had burning inside from the first day I had started this journey. My coach and friends now believed I just might accomplish what I wanted, and my family had always believed in me—but the judges—well, I didn't know what they believed. All I did know was they were the ones who gave me my scores, and I had yet to break a 9.0.

As a result, I shifted this deep desire to succeed from its former aim—proving to my coach and my friends that they were wrong about how good I could be—to changing the opinions of the judges who gave me my scores. My goal for the rest of the season would be to force the judges to give me higher scores because my performance would be so much better than everyone else's that they would have no other choice.

I was now down to three or four weeks before the end of the season, and I was not about to let someone else take something away from me that I thought I had earned. There was no more time left to make any major changes; there was just time enough to work on the little things, those things that separated the good from the great and the great from the best. My performance would need to be flawless, and if that was what it was going to take, then so be it. Win or lose, reach my goal or not, I was coming out swinging. I had not come this far to give anything less than 100 percent. I refused to have to look myself in the mirror, after everything was said and done, and know I hadn't given everything I could—no way, no how! That judge was going to have to take what I wanted away from me, and I would be damned if I wasn't going to make it harder than hell for him to do that!

That was my mind-set during my training and in competitions all through those last few stages of the season.

• *Chapter 18* •

The Outcome Says It All

Final Tests

The final tests for me would start with the Des Plaines Valley League Conference meet. Remember, it was last season at this time that I had seen Tom Ware perform, and he had won the meet. (Tom had graduated the year before and received an athletic scholarship to Northern Illinois University.) I certainly did not place in the top half of this competition the previous season; in fact, I was probably much closer to the bottom of the heap. However, so much had changed in the past year that I went into the meet feeling very confident.

There were not a lot of strong ringmen in the conference, which eased some of the pressure. There were a couple of very good teams, but rings, like pommel horse, is one of the more difficult events and there really wasn't anyone else capable of scoring in the nines. Of course, I knew full well that anything could happen. I had learned to never—and I mean NEVER—take anything for granted.

My high school hosted the conference this year, and I enjoyed competing in front of a home crowd. I was the last performer for my team on this event and felt that my performance had been good. (Of course, I *never* felt everything went perfectly, as I consistently dissected my routine with my brother and always seemed to come up with areas to improve.) My score was a 9.05! It was my first nine of the season—in fact, it was my first nine EVER. I won the meet, and the second-place competitor came in at 8.4, more than six-tenths of a point below me.

In the gymnastics world, six-tenths is a pretty big margin. I felt very good about this, but I was also very aware that the toughest competitors were going to come from other conferences. I would see them in the district, sectional, and state meets, if I made it that far. Everything at this point was now single elimination, meaning you would be eliminated from the state series at the point your performance failed to meet the criteria for moving on in this series. If you did not place in the top five in the district meet and the top three at the sectional meet, the only way you could still qualify into the state meet would be "at large." The numerous district meets funnel the best gymnasts into several sectionals around the state. After all district meets are completed, they combine all the scores from each meet, on each event. Beyond the top *five* gymnasts from each district who have already qualified, they also take those with the next nine highest scores, and these gymnasts are said to qualify at large to the sectional. The same process is used at the sectional competitions. The top twelve scores beyond the top *three* qualifiers from each sectional, on each event, qualify at large to compete in the one state meet. If you miss making it into either of these groups, at any time, you are done.

The district meet provided lots of competition. There were a lot of good gymnasts on rings competing here, and I would have to do well to move on to sectionals. The competition went smoothly and again, I felt my routine was good. I won the meet, but this time my score was an 8.85 and the next competitor was three-tenths away at 8.55. This is still a good margin; however, once again I did not break nine, and I felt I had competed just as well as I had in the conference meet.

I talked this over with my brother, and he felt the same way. I knew my performance was not perfect and that I always would find areas to improve in, but to us, both of these performances were very consistent. I discussed this with my coach, and he told me that as you continue on in the state series, the scoring would get tougher. Great! I had only scored in the nines once this season, and my coach was telling me it was going to get tougher? Man, I thought, he has got to be kidding; can't I ever get a break? My coach's explanation, even though accurate, was not acceptable to me. You might as well have put a bulls-eye on those judges' backs. I resented them, and again, this fueled more focused and determined training on my part, if that was possible. I would take care of this in the gym.

Within no time the sectional meet was here, and it was going to be intense. The athletes contending were not just good; they were excellent. Competition would be very tight. I remember for the first time being intimidated as I watched some of the gymnasts executing their skills during warm-ups. They really performed their swinging movements well, and several had strength combinations to match. I would definitely be challenged here. And, for the first time this season, I was truly "scared" of the competition and put a lot of pressure on myself. I knew how well I would need to do to win this meet, and I *had* to win, didn't I?

Perhaps needless to say, my routine was not as good as the two previous meets (conference and districts). Don't get me wrong—it was still good, but it was just that I was not as solid as before. You know—the little things! And guess what, they made a difference! I scored an 8.7 and took second place (good enough to qualify for state, but not good enough to win). Barry Schmidt, a ringman from Oak Park/River Forest, took first with a score of 9.0. This was the first time I had seen him compete. He was a big kid with an equally big swing. He looked good when he swung to a handstand and had only minor deductions for wobble when he got there. The rest of his routine was polished, and he performed a more difficult dismount than most, including mine. Best I had seen all season, and he deserved to beat me! At this meet, on this night, he was a full three-tenths better.

By the way, the third-place finisher scored an 8.55, only one-and-one-half-tenths lower than my score—I only became aware of this later, through the review of old newspaper clippings. I had learned in the past year to only concern myself with what lay before me, not behind me. As far as I was concerned, what was behind me was irrelevant. This is an important concept for any competitive athlete to learn. (There would be another very important principle I would learn, but that would not happen until the state meet.)

THE STATE MEET

My training before the state meet went very well. I continued per-fecting my skills by trying to be as explosive and solid as possible. I would not give up, and I continued demanding and accepting only the best from myself, keeping in mind that I had lost to someone for the first time this season (and rightfully so) and I had yet to compete against Bart Conner, future Olympian, World Champion and Gold Medalist, as well as several other excellent ringmen. And there were several sectional meets and many ringmen within these sectionals that I had yet to see compete. All of them would be at state, and only the best would get into the top ten for the finals. This I knew full well. Any mistake at this point would mean defeat. Mere tenths or hundredths of a point could determine the winner.

The atmosphere at the state meet was kind of crazy. Gymnasts, coaches, and judges were all over the competitive floor. Not only were the best gymnasts in the state here along with everyone else who had qualified, but the crowd of spectators was growing larger by the minute. I had never been here before, even to watch, and my coach and I were the only ones on the gym floor from my high school, as no one else from my team had made it into the state meet. I did have some friends in the stands and, of course, my family, but that was pretty much it.

My whole family was very supportive of my efforts—especially my father and brother, who never missed a meet. My dad had been out of work for eight months, and it was good to see him there. He had really been an inspiration to me. His belief in me had helped me develop my belief in myself, and now the possibility of achieving my goal was real. Who would have thought, a year ago on this day, that I would be standing here competing at this meet?

My warm-ups went well and I felt ready. All my hard work would come down to about a forty-five-second routine—hopefully two forty-five-second routines, but I would have to do well in the preliminary round to make it to the finals, and that was where my fo-cus was. (During competitions, I never thought past the task at hand. Considering or mulling over future events are really only good for planning training sessions, not competing.) If my recollection serves me correctly, I got a decent draw (placement of my turn among the group of gymnasts). I would compete somewhere in the middle. As far as I was concerned, the more competitors who went before me, the better. I loved seeing what I had to do—in other words, the performances that I had to top. Some people don't like this kind of pressure, but I loved it. If I had a choice, I would always go dead last.

About fifteen minutes before I competed, I went back into the warm-up gym to settle down. I performed parts of my routine to stay physically ready, and mentally I visualized each skill done perfectly. This was a ritual for me, and I did it consistently each time I competed, before I walked out to the main floor.

When my coach came to get me, I was nervous but focused (I always felt this way). We walked out together, and I remember how crowded the competitive floor was. There were the judges (two of them) and the gymnasts competing, or waiting to compete, along with their coaches, for all six events. In the preliminaries, all events ran simultaneously. I walked over to the rings, put chalk on my hands, and prepared to go.

My routine felt very good. Everything was smooth and solid, and I only took one step on my dismount (for me this was normal). I thought it was the best routine I had done all season, and so did my brother. My score was 8.95. This was a good score—but not good enough. It put me in second place, tied with Bart Conner, and just under two-tenths lower than Barry Schmidt's score of 9.1. I had made it into the finals, but felt as if everything was slipping away. I had performed the best I thought I could. I did not know what to think. I went over to my brother, and we talked. He also could not figure out what I was doing wrong that was keeping me out of the nines. How was I going to beat that kid from Oak Park?

I was disappointed, and my coach knew it. He came over to me and told me not to worry; the finals would start from scratch. Everyone in the top ten, or in this case eleven, because of my tie with Bart, would have a chance to win. We all started from zero. This made me feel a little better, but I still did not see any way of besting my previous performance. I could not stop trying to figure out what Schmidt was doing better than I was. He had already beaten me twice.

I went home that night somewhat depressed. I really was not sure what to think or do; there were so many thoughts going through my head. Yet through all of this, something stood out. It was a principle I had been learning and building on all season long but had temporarily forgotten. In both situations where I had lost, some of my focus or attention was on my competition. I was intimidated and challenged at sectionals and took second, and at state prelims I was competing against that same ringman along with several other very good competitors. The more I thought about this, the more I realized I was focusing on aspects over which I had no control—the other competitors! I thought I had known better than this, but this situation was a very clear reminder. I did not have control over what any other competitor did or did not do; I only had control over what I did. In that, I had complete control, and that was all that mattered.

From this point forward, I chose to focus only on what I needed to do. This made everything else irrelevant. Talk about relief! This focus took a lot of pressure off me. It was almost as if someone had lifted an anvil off my chest. That night I did some extra conditioning exercises for my straight-arm work, visualizing the whole time how I wanted these skills to be performed. I believed that my straight-arm work, along with my strength combinations, were my strong points, and tomorrow, in the finals, they would be at their peak. No matter what happened, I would give it my very best effort, focusing only on what I could control. Win or lose, I would be happy with myself.

I went to bed after my exercises and slept very well that night.

THE FINALS

I remember being very quiet and relaxed on the way to the finals. Choosing to focus only on what I had control over had a very calming effect. I had done everything that I could. No one I knew had more desire or had put in more time and effort than I had the past year, and this was also comforting.

When I got to the school and entered the gym, I noticed that I had been drawn to compete seventh in a field of eleven. My coach was very happy with the draw. It was not last, but it was close—and you know what? From my new perspective, it did not matter anyway! The real advantage of being able to compete later in the draw centered on the subjective gymnastics scoring system. Gymnastic scores tended to rise as more competitors went. This my coach knew very well.

I proceeded to the locker room to change and prepare for warm-ups. After dressing, I picked up my equipment bag and headed back to the gym. Finding an area to stretch out, I placed my bag behind me and began stretching while putting on my wrist-bands and grips (hand guards that give a gymnast a better grip on the apparatus). Once I felt ready, I went over to the chalk bin, put chalk on my hands, and waited my turn in line to jump up on the rings to continue preparing for the meet. I went through my normal event warm-up rituals, as I always had, and I remember feeling very strong—stronger than in the prelim warm-ups.

The gym was getting pretty crowded now. It seemed as if every school that had competitors in the meet brought their whole high school with them for support. Having a likely future Olympian, Bart Conner, in the meet undoubtedly brought a lot of media attention as well. And I had thought it was crowded in the prelims! That was nothing compared to the finals. It was standing room only, and in addition to the spectators, there were cameras and reporters all over

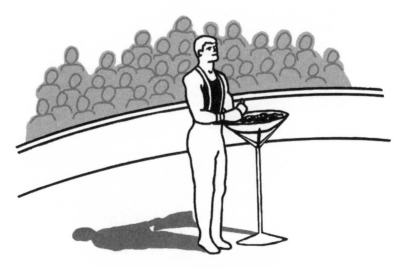

18.1: Preparation: "The Chalk Bin"

the place. Most of my friends had also come to see me compete. What a great atmosphere for the state finals!

Something else I became aware of, as I made my way through the competition floor and around the crowd, was that there did seem to be a real sense of support for me from students of other schools and from other spectators. This was most likely due to the fact that I was the only competitor from my high school in the state meet, let alone the finals, and they probably saw me as an "underdog." Most everyone else had other teammates on the floor with them.

Once the meet started, things settled down a little bit. The format in the finals was much different from in the prelims. Each event would be run separately instead of all at once. This would give all spectators, reporters, and coaches the opportunity to see every routine. The still rings would be the last event to go.

I spent most of my time going back and forth from the warm-up gym to the competitive floor, trying to determine when it would be best to start my final preparations. The meet ran smoothly, and before long, it was time for my event. I started my final warm-up and asked my coach to tell me when the gymnast who competed right before me was about to begin. When this occurred, my coach came in to get me. I finished with a couple of handstands on the floor, visualizing that solid feeling I wanted on the rings. I put on my team jacket and proceeded to the main floor. I noticed my family sitting in the middle of the stands off to the right of the still ring event. I looked up at them; they looked back. My dad was sweating bullets. (Was it nervousness, or the heat? It *was* warm in the gym!)

As the current competitor neared the end of his performance, I removed my jacket and made my way to the chalk bin. The chalk felt cool to the touch as I spread a thick layer on my hands and looked up again at my father. He seemed so proud of me but looked very nervous (it wasn't until years later that he told me how sick with anxiety he used to get when he watched me compete).

I remember thinking how much my dad had inspired me those many months ago, how much he had supported me in my endeavor, and how tough a year he had had, through being out of work for so long, and I distinctly remember wanting very much to win this championship for him. Not because he asked me or ever indicated such, but just because of who he was.

It was at that moment the competitor on the still rings landed his dismount, and my coach and I waited for the judges to complete his scores.

As I finished chalking up I tried to visualize a perfect performance in my head. This always helped me feel mentally prepared. The scores came up for the previous competitor, and it was time. I took one last look up at the stands directly at my brother. I put my fist over my heart and tapped. It would take the best performance of my life to win this thing; it would take "heart." There was nothing else to be said. My brother knew what I meant—he always did.

I turned my attention to the rings and walked over to the mat underneath them. It was so quiet you could hear a pin drop. That was amazing, considering the number of people in this gym. I looked toward the head judge, raised my hand, and he gave me the green flag. I focused my attention on the rings as my coach prepared to lift me up. I let them swing back once, then forward once, and on the back swing, I jumped and grabbed the rings, adjusting my grip until it felt right (this was all part of my own little ritual). My coach made sure I was still, and I started my performance. It was at that moment that everything seemed to slow down. It was as if I was there, but really not there, as though my mind and body were separate, yet completely in tune with each other. I was acutely aware of every movement of every muscle in my body and every movement of the rings, but I could still see everything around me.

My first skill was solid as a nail with no wobble, and so was the second. I remember thinking how good it felt to perform these two movements in this manner. (Now *that* is what I call fun!) They seemed effortless, and the rings were dead still upon their completion—that was a good thing! I moved into the strength portion of my routine, and again, it felt very easy to do. I looked out into the gym and saw hands moving together but could not hear a thing. It was almost as if I was deaf. I finished up this sequence, pressed up to a handstand, and powered back down into my final strength move. Again it felt effortless and amazingly, still no sound. I noticed that my body and the rings were, again, perfectly still, and I remember saying to myself, "I must stick my dismount."

As I finished up my routine and started my double, I stayed focused on where my body was in the air in relation to the floor. I saw the floor spin by once, then twice, and when I sensed the time was right I opened from my double. I tried to relax a little in my legs as I landed, and as I hit the ground, I felt balanced right over the top of my feet. No movement. Well, that was a first! I had never stuck my dismount this solid before. I almost always took one little step. I raised my hands to salute the judge, then dropped my arms and turned my attention up toward my family. They were all standing with arms raised in the air and applauding. It felt good, really good. At that moment, it did not matter whether I won or lost. That was not up to me. All I knew was I had just performed the best routine of my life. I really had thought I could not beat yesterday's performance, but I had—or at least I believed I had—and that was all that mattered.

My coach and I waited for my scores. This seemed to take forever. When my average score was finally raised I was shocked: a 9.25! This put me in first place with only four competitors left. It was also the third-highest score on this event in state meet history! Things looked good.

The next four competitors went, and none of them equaled or bettered my score. I had won, and not just by a little. The second place score was a 9.0 tie between two other very good ringmen, Carl Olsen from Glenbrook South and Greg Dreher from Reavis High School. I had won by over two-tenths of a point and scored in the nines! Barry Schmidt from Oak Park scored an 8.95 and ended up in a tie for fourth with Gary Rust from York. Bart Conner, from Niles West, tied for sixth place with Breck Grigas (future National Team Member) from Hinsdale Central, with a score of 8.9.

My coach congratulated me with a pat on the back. I had done it.

I walked up to the awards stand and shook hands with everyone. I stepped up on the first-place stand, shook the meet director's hand, and received the first-place medal. I looked up in the stands at my family and noticed tears running down my father's face. It had been a rough year for him, and my accomplishment made him proud and emotional. I thought to myself, "Dad, that was for you."

THE SCHOLARSHIP

After the meet, Chuck Ehrlich, the head coach from Northern Illinois University, talked with me about competing for him next season. NIU would be one of three universities that would eventually seriously recruit me; my choice was NIU. Tom Ware competed for Northern Illinois and had placed in the top ten at the NCAA Division I National Championships his freshman year on still rings. There was no way I would miss a chance to compete with him.

Amazing how one moment in a person's life can cause such a profound change. One year before this, I was a complete unknown whose name no one even knew. Who would have predicted I'd make over three-points improvement in about a year, win a state championship, and earn a full-ride scholarship to Northern Illinois University to compete for the Huskies? Certainly not anyone with any common sense.

Many have said that I must have been extremely talented to accomplish this in such a short period of time, but they are mistaken. What I did had very little to do with talent, but *everything* to do with my own, self-determined choices. I was no more talented than anyone else I competed against. In fact, I believe that although all of us are born with strengths and/or tendencies to excel in certain areas, the key for any person who wants to achieve success is to find out where his or her talents lie and then, most important, *commit themselves to making the right choices*—choices about goals, choices as to how to proceed toward them, choices about how much work it is going to take, and choices to go after the goal wholeheartedly and without hesitance or reservation. It is these choices that will ultimately make the difference between success and failure. The difference is in the individual's own *choice*, not necessarily his or her *talent*.

★ ★ ★

I have shared my story here so you can see in detail how this worked out in my own situation and what it took for me to excel in my chosen gymnastics event. In my case, no one could seriously claim that I was talented all along and would have had it made, no matter what. That was simply not true.

· Chapter 19 ·

When All Is Said and Done

Conclusion

$\mathcal{A}$s I stated earlier, my early athletic experiences had a profound effect on my life. They set me upon a path many are afraid to travel. My purpose here has been to share with you the knowledge, concepts, and principles I learned during my journey and make it easier for you. If, through my efforts, I am able to inspire at least one person to reach beyond their own present limits and make the effort to achieve something that many see as impossible, then what I have done was not in vain.

I want you to realize one of the most valuable things that anyone could ever teach you: that your true destiny lies in your own hands, and that this destiny has much more to do with the choices you make than with the talent you currently possess. It would be deeply satisfying to me to have had some part in helping you accomplish levels of performance that others only dream of.

Please keep in mind that no one can ever guarantee athletic success, just like there are no guarantees in life generally. All any person can do is lay out as many "chips" in their favor as possible. Hopefully, the information in this book will help you with this objective, so that someday you can look in the mirror and say to yourself, "I like who I am, what I've become, and who I plan to be." It is this statement that brings with it the truest sense of happiness and well-being.

I'd also like to leave you with an idea—sort of a prediction—which you are entirely free to agree with or reject, as you wish. This will be more true for some and perhaps less true for others. As you progress in your chosen sport, you might discover that your greatest satisfaction (self-satisfaction) is coming not necessarily from your accomplishments and wins, but from your willingness to go through the process and from everything that comes out of this process. You will begin to discover what I mean by "everything that comes out of this process" yourself, as you progress. But it has a lot to do with the fact that much of the real and lasting value of athletic endeavor is intrinsic; it comes from within yourself as you work toward the fulfillment of your goals. You might look at these intrinsic values as side benefits, but sometimes they prove to be what it was *all* about, after all—something much greater and more valuable to you even than athletics. This is the magic of athletic endeavor: by offering a path to personal fulfillment far greater than you might ever expect, it can transcend life itself.

Who Am I?

The Libero Code

— **Who am I?** A question best answered first by stating who I am not. I am not the point scorer on the team with massive hitting and blocking potential. I do not look over the net or down at my opponents when I jump. I am not the quarterback who runs our plays or decides who will get the next kill. It is very unlikely that you will ever read my name in the headlines of the newspaper or hear the crowd roar in awe over my performance. It is not the media, nor the spectators, nor even the college recruiters who will notice me first. To me, this is irrelevant anyway, for they are not the reason I play.

— **Who am I?** Well, our opponents will know who I am. Their hitters will fear me, their setters will run plays away from me, and their servers will try to avoid me. Our opponents may make what looks like an awesome play, but I will be there—waiting and watching, focused, and planning my next movement based on what is happening on the court. I am quick, I am fast, and I am very determined. If it is asked of me, I will deliver. Any opening that may appear will only be there for an instant because my job, my expectation, will be to fill that void.

— **Who am I?** I am the player who starts almost every offensive play. I cannot play poorly, EVER, because if I do, my setter will have a tough day and my hitters will not get their kills, and my team will not win. Then no one gets their name in the paper.

— **Who am I?** I am the player who gets very little credit for any of our wins and may get much of the blame for our losses. But, you know what? I would not have it any other way. That is the expectation for my position. My teammates know my role and my overall importance to our success, and that is what really counts.

— **Who am I?** I am the player warning all opponents who step onto our court to bring their A game because that is what I will bring every day, in every game, and for every point. If any opponent beats my team, be forewarned: we will be back, and I will be better than when you saw me the first time. Make no mistake—when I am on the court you will truly be in a battle—a war. I will give my heart, my soul, and my body for my team. If you want to beat us you will have to take the game from us, and you will have to go through me to do it. My plan is to make the time you spend on the court against my team very short.

— **Who am I?** I am your worst nightmare, and you need to be aware of the fact that I am not afraid. I relish the competition and the challenge that you place before me. Why? Because the court is mine. I own it from the first serve to the last hit you will make.

— **Who am I?** I am the Defensive Specialist, the Libero,[1] and you will never forget the impact I had on our match.

Your Greatest Gift to Yourself

The power to become whatever and whomever you decide, and the realization that you actually have this power, is one of the greatest gifts you can give to yourself.

References and Notes

CHAPTER 1

1. Bethany Hamilton's biographical information is from the website, Bethany, at http://bethanyhamilton.com/about/bio/ (accessed 2010).

CHAPTER 2

1. Norman L. Macht, *Jim Abbott* (New York: Chelsea House Publishers, 1994), 13, 19, and 26.

2. Jim Abbott's team information is from the website Baseball-reference .com, http://www.baseballreference.com/a/abbotji01.shtml (accessed April 20, 2006).

3. The 20th Century Awards, "SI's Top 10 Sports Moments of the 20th Century," December 3, 1999, http://sportsillustrated.cnn.com/features/cover/news/1999/12/02/awards/ (accessed November 14, 2011).

CHAPTER 3

1. Jim MacLaren's biographical information is courtesy of Jim MacLaren and his surviving sister, Jennifer Hippensteel; certain information

obtained from his website, with permission, at http://www.jimmaclaren
.com/ (accessed December 2008).

2. George Bernard Shaw, *Mrs. Warren's Profession,* Act II (1893), re-
printed on the website The Quotations Page, http://www.quotationspage
.com/quote/26793.html (accessed July 20, 2011).

3. Amy Ruth, *Wilma Rudolph* (Minneapolis, MN: Lerner Publications
Company, 2000), pp. 8–9, 15–19, 22–23; Corinne J. Naden, *Wilma Rudolph* (Chicago: Raintree, 2003), pp. 7, 9–15, 44–46.

4. Corinne J. Naden, *Wilma Rudolph* (Chicago: Raintree, 2003), p. 7.

CHAPTER 4

1. "The Legend, the Legacy, the Lessons, the Life of Coach John R.
Wooden," The John R. Wooden Course website, at http://www.wooden
course.com/who_is_john_wooden.html (accessed July 20, 2011).

2. Naismith Memorial Basketball Hall of Fame, http://www.hoophall
.com/hall-of-famers-index/ (accessed July 20, 2011).

3. John Wooden and Steve Jamison, *My Personal Best: Life Lessons from
an All-American Journey* (New York: The McGraw-Hill Companies, 2004),
p. xi.

4. "Pyramid of Success," The Official Site of Coach John Wooden,
http://www.coachwooden.com/index2.html (accessed July 20, 2011).

5. John Wooden and Steve Jamison, *My Personal Best: Life Lessons from
an All-American Journey* (New York: The McGraw-Hill Companies, 2004),
pp. xi–xiii, 1–9, 90.

6. "Former Players Remember Coach Wooden," *Los Angeles Wave,*
June 5, 2010, http://www.wavenewspapers.com/sports/95710689.html
(accessed July 29, 2011).

CHAPTER 5

1. Merriam-Webster, m-w.com (Springfield, MA: Merriam-Webster,
Incorporated), http://www.merriam-webster.com/dictionary/character
(accessed August 2011).

2. Elizabeth J. Jewell and Frank Abate, eds., *The New Oxford American
Dictionary* (New York: Oxford University Press, Inc., 2001), p. 882.

CHAPTER 6

1. Josh Alper, "Sorting Out Jose Canseco on Steroids," video interview of May 7, 2009, Jose Canseco press conference, NBC Chicago, May 8, 2009, at http://www.nbcchicago.com/news/sports/Sorting-Out-Jose -Canseco.html (accessed July 20, 2011).

2. Christine Hauser and Ben Shpigel, "Baseball Announces Steroids Investigation," March 30, 2006, NYTimes.com, http://www.nytimes. com/2006/03/30/sports/baseball/31cnd-base.html (accessed April 2006); Associated Press, "Baseball to Investigate Bonds, Other Players: Selig Hires ex-Senator Leader Mitchell in Wake of BALCO Case, New Book," NBS Sports, MSNBC, http://www.msnbc.msn.com/id/12070797/ (accessed April 2006).

3. George J. Mitchell, "Report to the Commissioner of Baseball of an Independent Investigation into the Illegal Use of Steroids and Other Performance Enhancing Substances by Players in Major League Baseball," DLA Piper US, LLP (December 13, 2007): SR-1.

4. Bonnie D. Ford, "Landis Admits Doping, Accuses Lance," ESPN Cycling and BMX, May 21, 2010, http://sports.espn.go.com/oly/cycling/ news/story?id=5203604 (accessed July 22, 2011).

5. ESPN.com News Services, "Source: Cushing Test Flagged hCG," ESPN NFL, May 10, 2010, http://sports.espn.go.com/nfl/news/ story?id=5176949 (accessed July 22, 2011).

6. "A Summary of the Sports Illustrated Lance Armstrong Investigation," *Cycling News*, Second Edition, January 19, 2011, http://www .cyclingnews.com/news/a-summary-of-the-sports-illustrated-lance -armstrong-investigation (accessed July 22, 2011).

7. Rob Gloster, "Regina Jacobs Suspended for Four Years for Steroid Use." USAToday.com, Olympics section, July 17, 2004.

8. Associated Press, "Ex-Olympian Tim Montgomery Pleads Guilty in Multimillion-Dollar Fraud Scheme" FoxNews.com, U.S. section, April 10, 2007, http://www.foxnews.com/story/0,2933,264956,00. html (accessed October 2007); Associated Press, "Montgomery Is Sentenced," *New York Times*, Sports Briefing/Track and Field section, May 17, 2008, http://query.nytimes.com/gst/fullpage.html?res=9A03EEDD 1231F934A25756C0A96E9C8B63&ref=timmontgomery (accessed July 21, 2011).

9. Associated Press, "Montgomery Sentenced to 5 Years," New York Times, More Sports section, October 10, 2008, http://www.nytimes

.com/2008/10/11/sports/othersports/11montgomery.html?adxnnl=1&
adxnnlx=1322316764-jqvZctjqz1Wb8sOOQqzIzA (accessed July 22, 2011).

10. Amy Shipley, "Marion Jones Admits to Steroid Use," In the News section, *Washington Post*, October 5, 2007, http://www.washingtonpost.com/wp-dyn/content/article/2007/10/04/AR2007100401666.html (accessed July 21, 2011).

11. Dr. Charles E. Yesalis and Dr. Michael S. Bahrke, "Anabolic-Androgenic Steroids: Incidence of Use and Health Implications," President's Council on Physical Fitness and Sports *Research Digest*, Series 5, No. 5, March 2005, http://www.fitness.gov/Digest-March2005.pdf (accessed July 2011). Dr. Yesalis has testified before the U.S. Congress on many occasions regarding the use of performance-enhancing drugs in elite sports (high-level amateur athletics at the high school, college, and Olympic levels) and by children. He has also studied the incidence of AS use among elite power lifters, college athletes, and professional football players. In 1993, using nationwide data, he demonstrated the association between AS use and violent behavior. He also showed that there is an association between AS use and the use of other illicit drugs and alcohol.

12. T. R. Reid, "Rape Case against Bryant Is Dropped, Accuser Decided against Testifying," *Washington Post*, Postsports section, September 2, 2004, http://www.washingtonpost.com/wp-dyn/articles/A52941-2004Sep1.html (accessed July 23, 2011).

13. Joe Mandak, "Judge Sides with Michael Jordan against Woman Who Claims He Fathered Her Child," KingsFans.com, Sports–NBA section, April 11, 2008, http://www.kingsfans.com/forums/showthread.php?26814-The-Michael-Jordan-Paternity-suit.....-ugh.. (accessed July 24, 2011).

14. Russell Goldman, "At Least 9 Women Linked to Tiger Woods in Alleged Affairs," ABC News, Entertainment section, December 7, 2009, http://abcnews.go.com/Entertainment/tiger-woods-women-linked-alleged-affairs/story?id=9270076#.TsLzdvEyGas (accessed July 23, 2011).

CHAPTER 7

1. FOX Sports, NewsCore section, "Wrestler with One Leg Wins NCAA Title," March 19, 2011, http://msn.foxsports.com/other/story/Anthony-Robles-wrestler-with-one-leg-wins-national-title-031911 (accessed July 23, 2011).

CHAPTER 12

1. Plyometrics trains the muscles for speed and explosiveness (power). This is done by loading the muscle with energy through stretching (called an "eccentric" contraction), immediately followed by a tightening of that same muscle (called a "concentric" contraction). Jumping down from a box then immediately jumping back up would be a good example of a plyometric-type movement for the legs.

CHAPTER 15

1. IHSA refers to the Illinois High School Association.

WHO AM I?: THE LIBERO CODE

1. A libero is a designated back-row defensive player in volleyball. Specific rules govern the actions of a libero.

Index

Abbott, Jim (baseball pitcher), 30, 35, 57, 84
adversity as motivation, 40–43
Armstrong, Lance (cyclist), 73
athletic codes. *See* codes of conduct
attitudes of athletes: "all work and no play," 54; arrogance of athletes, 3; influence of support-givers on, 2; toward competitors, 109–11; "What's in it for me?" 3. *See also* mind-set for achievement

Bahrke, Michael S., 77
baseball: pitcher in training, 103–5; steroid use, 63, 71–73
basketball, training, 128–29
Beamon, Bob (Olympic long jumper), 91
Becoming a True Champion (Mango and Lamont), xii, 4
Bonds, Barry (baseball player), 72
boxing, conditioning program, 147–48
Bryant, Kobe (basketball player), 77–78

Canseco, Jose (baseball player), 71–72
CDSPH (Commitment, Discipline, Sacrifice, Priorities, Heart) Principle, 51–60; taking action exercises, 59–60

character and integrity, 61–68; athletic codes and, 64–67; in athletics today, 62–64; character defined, 61; consequences of cheating on, 79–80; developing, 3, 6, 64; integrity defined, 62
cheating, 69–81; consequences of, 79–80; defined, 69; physical consequences of drug use, 78–79; prevalence in sports, 71–76; sex scandals in sports, 77–79; steroid use in sports, 63, 71–75; taking action exercise, 80–81
circle of achievement (COA), 157–68; advanced skills and technical elements, 160, 172; conditioning elements, 161, 173; fundamentals, 159, 171; gymnastics training example, 164–66; mental and emotional elements, 161; taking action exercise, 167–68; volleyball training example, 161–64; worksheets, 169–74
circle of success, 84
club jumping, 21
coaches: accountability for team performance, 18; criticism of, 19; training and guidance role, 20

233

About the Authors

Kirk Mango was a collegiate Division I national champion and gold medalist on the still rings in 1979; he defeated several Olympians to earn this honor. The previous year Kirk had won the silver medal on this event in the 1978 Division I National Championships. He was selected as a collegiate All-American in both 1978 and 1979, and to the present day he still holds the Northern Illinois University school record for the still rings event. Kirk is also a three-time Hall of Fame athlete and was selected in 2009 as Number 8 on the list of "Top 50 Huskies of All Time" by the NIU *Northern Star*. He has been a high school teacher for thirty-two years, coaching for seventeen of them. He has coached girls' gymnastics teams to three conference championships, four regional championships, one sectional championship, and three Elite-Eight IHSA (Illinois High School Association) state championship competitions. In addition, Kirk writes and manages a popular blog, *The Athlete's Sports Experience: Making a Difference,* on the ChicagoNow blog network. His articles have also appeared on the Gatorade Moms and Weplay Moms sports websites.

Daveda Lamont has coauthored three nonfiction books; additionally, her historical Native American novella, *The Way of the Eagle: An Early California Journey of Awakening*, was published in 2011 and honored as a finalist in the visionary fiction category of the USA "Best Books 2011" awards, sponsored by USA Book News. A developmental editor and ghostwriter with many nonfiction books to her credit, she has also served as a contract editor for Powered, Inc., editing and cowriting courses for the corporate online universities of clients such as Barnes & Noble, Dell, Visa, and Bloomberg. com. Her editorial work has encompassed the subject areas of fine art appreciation, film and music instruction, celebrity/artist memoirs, creative nonfiction, nutrition/diet, alternative health care, family financial planning, consumer investing and finance, and self-improvement, among others.